Registered Health Information Technician (RHIT) Exam Preparation

Ninth Edition

Darcy Carter, DHSc, MHA, RHIA

Patricia Shaw, EdD, RHIA, FAHIMA

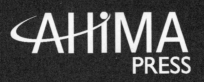

ISBN: 978-1-58426-872-7
eISBN: 978-1-58426-873-4

AHIMA Product No.: AB105022

AHIMA Staff:
Sarah Cybulski, MA, Assistant Editor
Megan Grennan, Director, Content Production and AHIMA Press
James Pinnick, Vice President, Content and Learning Solutions
Rachel Schratz, MA, Associate Digital Content Developer

Cover image: © 31moonlight31; iStock

For more information, including updates, about AHIMA Press publications, visit http://www.ahima.org/education/press.

American Health Information Management Association
233 North Michigan Avenue, 21st Floor
Chicago, Illinois 60601-5809
ahima.org

Contents

About the Editors

Darcy Carter, DHSc, MHA, RHIA, earned her doctorate degree in health science with an emphasis in leadership and organizational behavior and her master's degree in healthcare administration. Dr. Carter is currently department chair, associate professor, and MHA program director at Weber State University, where she teaches courses in coding, reimbursement, quality management, and healthcare management. Dr. Carter is also coauthor of *Quality and Performance Improvement in Healthcare: Theory, Practice, and Management* published by AHIMA.

Patricia Shaw, EdD, RHIA, FAHIMA, holds a doctorate and master's degree in education. She is currently professor emerita and adjunct professor at Weber State University, where she teaches quality and performance improvement and coding courses. Prior to her position at Weber State, Dr. Shaw managed hospital health information management services departments and was a nosologist for 3M Health Information Systems. Dr. Shaw is also coauthor of *Quality and Performance Improvement in Healthcare: Theory, Practice, and Management* published by AHIMA.

Acknowledgments

The authors and AHIMA Press would like to acknowledge Angela Campbell, MSHI, RHIA, FAHIMA, AHIMA-Approved ICD-10-CM/PCS Trainer, for her technical review of this text.

About the RHIT Exam

Professionals who hold the Registered Health Information Technician (RHIT) credential are health information technicians who ensure the quality of medical records by verifying their completeness, accuracy, and proper entry into computer systems. They may also use computer applications to assemble and analyze patient data for the purpose of improving patient care or controlling costs. RHITs often specialize in coding diagnoses and procedures in patient records for reimbursement and research.

Although most RHITs work in hospitals, you will also find them in a variety of other healthcare settings including office-based physician practices, nursing homes, home health agencies, mental health facilities, and public health agencies. In fact, employment opportunities exist for RHITs in any organization that uses patient data or health information, such as pharmaceutical companies, law and insurance firms, and health product vendors.

Detailed information about the RHIT exam and academic eligibility requirements can be found at http://www.ahima.org/certification.

The National Commission for Certifying Agencies (NCCA) has granted accreditation to AHIMA's RHIT certification program for demonstrating compliance with the NCCA Standards for the Accreditation of Certification Programs. NCCA is the accrediting body of the Institute for Credentialing Excellence (formerly the National Organization for Competency Assurance).

The NCCA Standards were created in 1977 and updated in 2014 to ensure certification programs adhere to modern standards of practice for the certification industry. AHIMA joins an elite group of more than 100 organizations representing more than 200 programs that have received and maintained NCCA accreditation. More information on the NCCA is available online at http://www.credentialingexcellence.org/ncca.

RHIT Exam Competency Statements

A certification exam is based on an explicit set of competencies. These competencies have been determined through a practitioners' job analysis study. The competencies are subdivided into domains and tasks, as listed here. The exam tests only content pertaining to these competencies. Each domain is allocated a predefined number of questions to make up the exam.

Domain 1: Data Content, Structure, and Information Governance (19–25%)

1. Apply health information guidelines (for example, coding guidelines, CMS, facility or regional best practices, federal and state regulations).
2. Apply healthcare standards (for example, Joint Commission, Meaningful Use).
3. Identify and maintain the designated record set.
4. Maintain the integrity of the health record (for example, identify and correct issues within the EHR).
5. Audit content and completion of the health record (for example, validate document content).
6. Educate clinicians on documentation and content.
7. Coordinate document control (for example, create, revise, standardize forms).
8. Assess and maintain the integrity of the master patient index (MPI).
9. Maintain and understand data workflow.

10. Create and maintain functionalities of the EHR.
11. Create and maintain EHR reports to ensure data integrity.
12. Navigate patient portals and provide education and support.

Domain 2: Access, Disclosure, Privacy, and Security (14–18%)

1. Manage the access, use, and disclosure of PHI using laws, regulations, and guidelines (for example, release of information, accounting of disclosures).
2. Determine right of access to the legal health record.
3. Educate internal and external customers (for example, clinicians, staff, volunteers, students, patients, insurance companies, attorneys) on privacy, access, and disclosure.
4. Apply record retention guidelines (for example, retain, archive, or destroy).
5. Mitigate privacy and security risk.
6. Identify and correct identity issues within the EHR (for example, merges, documentation corrections, registration errors, overlays).

Domain 3: Data Analytics and Use (11–18%)

1. Identify common internal and external data sources.
2. Extract data.
3. Analyze data.
4. Report patient data (for example, CDC, CMS, MACs, RACs, insurers).
5. Compile healthcare statistics and create reports, graphs, and charts.
6. Analyze common data metrics used to evaluate health information functions (for example, CMI, census productivity, CDI query rate, ROI turnaround time).

Domain 4: Revenue Cycle Management (19–25%)

1. Identify the components of the revenue cycle process.
2. Demonstrate proper use of clinical indicators to improve the integrity of coded data.
3. Code health record documentation.
4. Query clinicians to clarify documentation.
5. Recall utilization review processes and objectives.
6. Manage denials (for example, coding or insurance).
7. Conduct coding and documentation audits.
8. Provide coding and documentation education.
9. Monitor discharged, not final billed (DNFB).
10. Analyze the case mix.
11. Identify common billing issues for inpatient and outpatient.
12. Understand payer guidelines and requirements (for example, LCDs, NCDs, fee schedules, conditions of participation).
13. Collaborate with clinical documentation integrity (CDI) staff.
14. Review and maintain a charge description master (CDM).
15. Describe different payment methodologies and different types of health insurance plans (for example, public vs private).

Domain 5: Compliance (13–17%)

1. Perform quality assessments.
2. Monitor health information compliance and report noncompliance (for example, coding, ROI, CDI).
3. Maintain standards for health information functions (for example, chart completion, coding accuracy, ROI turnaround time, departmental workflow).
4. Monitor regulatory changes for timely and accurate implementation.

Domain 6: Leadership (9–12%)

1. Provide education regarding health information laws and regulations.
2. Review health information processes.
3. Develop and revise policies and procedures (for example, compliance, ROI, coding).
4. Establish standards for health information functions (for example, chart completion, coding accuracy, ROI, turnaround time, departmental workflow).
5. Collaborate with other departments for health information interoperability.
6. Provide health information subject matter expertise.
7. Understand the principles and guidelines of project management.

RHIT Exam Specifications

The RHIT exam lasts three and a half hours and is made up of 150 multiple choice questions. ICD-10-CM, ICD-10-PCS, CPT, and HCPCS coding concepts are tested; however, no code books are needed to take the RHIT exam. All necessary information needed to answer coding questions is included. During the exam, candidates are provided all of the appropriate information to answer a question on the exam. Therefore, commonly used hospital statistical formulas are provided if a question requires calculations that go beyond basic rates and percentages. These formulas are also listed in the back of this book. A calculator is available during the exam. For the most up-to-date RHIT exam information, visit http://ahima.org/certification.

How to Use This Book and Website

The *Registered Health Information Technician (RHIT) Exam Preparation* and accompanying website contain multiple choice practice questions and exams that test the knowledge of content pertaining to the RHIT competencies published by AHIMA.

The format presented in this exam prep is similar to the RHIT certification exam. This exam prep contains 550 multiple choice practice questions and two complete practice exams of 150 questions each that are organized by the RHIT domains. Because each question is identified by one of the six RHIT domains, you will be able to determine when checking your answers whether you need knowledge or skill building in a particular area of the exam domains. Pursuing answer references will then help you to build knowledge and skills in specific domains.

To effectively use this book, work through the practice questions first. This approach will help you to identify areas in which you may need further preparation by checking your answers against the answer key afterwards. For the questions that you answer incorrectly, read the associated reference material to refresh your knowledge. After going through the practice questions, take one of the practice exams. Again, for the questions that you answer incorrectly, refresh your knowledge by reading the associated reference material. Continue in the same manner with the second exam.

The accompanying website contains the same 550 practice questions and the two practice exams that are printed in the book. Each of the self-scoring exams can be run in practice mode, which allows you to work at your own pace; or exam mode, which simulates the three and a half hour timed exam experience. The practice questions and simulated exams online can be presented in random order, or you may choose to go through the questions in sequential order by domains. You may also choose to practice or test your skills on specific domains. For example, if you would like to enhance your skills in domain 2, you may choose only domain 2 questions for a given practice session. You may retake the practice exams as many times as you like.

Study Tips

The best way to prepare for the RHIT Certification Exam is to study the material you have learned over the course of your health information technology educational program. It is difficult to remember everything you have learned over the course of the program, so it is important to review the information. Study is the best way to prepare for the exam. Carefully review the information in the Commission on Certification for Health Informatics and Information Management Candidate Guide. You will want to prepare yourself mentally, physically, and emotionally to succeed.

Tips while studying:
- Get enough sleep.
- Eat a healthy, well-balanced diet.
- Stay hydrated.
- Take breaks.
- Exercise.
- Don't try to memorize everything, work at understanding.
- Use tricks to remember the material, like using an acronym or another type of association.
- Eliminate other stressors, as much as possible.
- Take a practice exam in the three and a half hour time frame you will have for the exam.
- If you do not know where the testing center is located, visit it before the day of the exam. This will help you avoid getting lost or being late for your exam.

Exam Day Tips

- Get enough sleep in the days leading up to the exam.
- Wear clothes that you are comfortable in and dress in layers so you can remove or add a layer depending on the temperature of the exam room.
- Eat a nutritious breakfast.
- Allow yourself enough time to get ready to leave so you are not rushed.
- Arrive at the testing center 30 minutes prior to your exam time.
- Bring the required identification.
- You will have three and a half hours to complete the exam. Do not obsess over the clock in the room but do budget your time. This should allow you to answer each question and review any questions you may have not answered because you wanted to come back to them.
- Time management will be an important part of taking the exam.
- Read each question carefully. Do not automatically assume you know the answer to a question without first carefully reading the entire question and each answer choice carefully. After reviewing each answer choice, choose the best answer.
- Skip and come back to any questions where you are unsure of the answer or the question is too difficult. You may find information in another question that will help you recall the answer to a question you skipped. Manage your time well while you do this.
- Do answer every test question. A guess is better than not answering a question at all; but, do so after carefully reviewing the question and the possible answers. After you eliminate the answers you know are incorrect, make the best choice. A true guess will give you a one-in-four chance of answering a question correctly.
- Relax as much as possible and BREATHE. You can do this!

PRACTICE EXAM 1

Domain 1 *Data Content, Structure, and Information Governance*

1. A new health information management (HIM) director has been asked by the hospital CIO to ensure data content standards are identified, understood, implemented, and managed for the hospital's EHR system. Which of the following should be the HIM director's first step in carrying out this responsibility?

    a. Call the EHR vendor and ask to review the system's data dictionary.

    b. Identify data content requirements for all areas of the organization.

    c. Schedule a meeting with all department directors to get their input.

    d. Review CMS guidelines to determine what data sets are required to be collected.

2. Standardizing medical terminology to avoid differences in naming various health conditions and procedures (such as the synonyms *bunionectomy*, *McBride procedure*, and *repair of hallux valgus*) is one purpose of:

    a. Content and structure standards

    b. Security standard

    c. Transaction standards

    d. Vocabulary standards

3. At admission, Mrs. Smith's date of birth is recorded as 3/25/1948. An audit of the EHR discovers that the numbers in the date of birth are transposed in reports. This situation reflects a problem in:

    a. Data comprehensiveness

    b. Data consistency

    c. Data currency

    d. Data granularity

4. Identify the documentation that records the attending physician's assessment of the patient's current health status.

    a. Physical examination

    b. Medical history

    c. Progress notes

    d. Discharge summary

5. Which of the following is a key characteristic of the problem-oriented health record?

    a. Allows all providers to document in the health record

    b. Uses laboratory reports and other diagnostic tools to determine health problems

    c. Provides electronic documentation in the health record

    d. Uses an itemized list of the patient's past and present health problems

6. A health record technician has been asked to review the discharge patient abstracting module of a proposed new electronic health record (EHR). Which of the following data sets would the technician consult to ensure the system collects all federally required discharge data elements for Medicare and Medicaid inpatients in an acute-care hospital?

   a. CARF

   b. DEEDS

   c. UACDS

   d. UHDDS

7. A health data analyst has been asked to compile a report of the percentage of patients who had a baseline partial thromboplastin time (PTT) test performed prior to receiving heparin. What clinical reports in the health record would the health data analyst need to consult in order to prepare this report?

   a. Physician progress notes and medication record

   b. Nursing and physician progress notes

   c. Medication administration record and clinical laboratory reports

   d. Physician orders and clinical laboratory reports

8. Which of the following is considered the authoritative resource in locating a health record?

   a. Disease index

   b. Master patient index

   c. Patient directory

   d. Patient registry

9. A family practitioner requests the opinion of a physician specialist who reviews the patient's health record and examines the patient. In what type of report would the physician specialist record findings, impressions, and recommendations?

   a. Consultation

   b. Medical history

   c. Physical examination

   d. Progress notes

10. The master patient index (MPI) manager has identified a pattern of duplicate health record numbers from the specimen processing area of the hospital. The MPI manager merged the patient information and corrected the duplicates in the patient information system. After this merging process, which department should the MPI manager notify to correct the source system data?

    a. Laboratory

    b. Radiology

    c. Quality Management

    d. Registration

11. What type of analysis compares omitted clinical information received from external providers with the needed clinical information to make a correct diagnosis?

    a. Risk management analysis

    b. Qualitative analysis

    c. Gap analysis

    d. Document management analysis

12. To comply with the Joint Commission standards, the HIM director wants to ensure the history and physical examinations are documented in the patient's health record no later than 24 hours after admission. Which of the following would be the best way to ensure the completeness of the health record?

    a. Establish a process to review health records immediately on discharge.

    b. Review each patient's health record concurrently to ensure the history and physicals are present.

    c. Retrospectively review each patient's health record to ensure the history and physicals are present.

    d. Write a memorandum to all physicians relating the Joint Commission requirements for documenting history and physical examinations.

13. The HIM director is having difficulty with the emergency services on-call physicians completing their health records. Currently, three deficiency notices are sent to the physicians through the EHR system including an initial notice, a second reminder, and a final notification. Which of the following would be the best first step in trying to rectify the current situation?

    a. Call the Joint Commission and notify them of noncompliant physicians.

    b. Consult with the medical director who has authority over the on-call physicians for suggestions on how to improve response to the current notices.

    c. Post the hospital policy in the emergency department.

    d. Routinely send out a fourth notice to remind each physician of his or her documentation obligations.

14. Creekside Care, a skilled nursing facility, wants to become certified to take part in federal government reimbursement programs such as Medicare and Medicaid. What standards must the facility meet to become certified for these programs?

    a. Minimum Data Set

    b. National Commission on Correctional Health Care

    c. Medicare Conditions of Participation

    d. Outcomes and Assessment Information Set

15. A health record with deficiencies that is not completed within the timeframe specified in the medical staff rules and regulations is called a(n):

    a. Suspended record

    b. Delinquent record

    c. Pending record

    d. Illegal record

16. How do accreditation organizations such as the Joint Commission use the health record?

    a. To serve as a source for case study information

    b. To determine whether the documentation supports the provider's claim for reimbursement

    c. To provide healthcare services

    d. To determine whether standards of care are being met

17. Which of the following specialized patient assessment tools must be used by Medicare-certified home care providers?

    a. Minimum data set for long-term care

    b. Outcomes and Assessment Information Set

    c. Patient assessment instrument

    d. Resident assessment protocol

18. Before healthcare organizations can provide services, they usually must obtain this from government entities such as the state or county in which they are located.

    a. Accreditation

    b. Certification

    c. Licensure

    d. Permission

19. The following descriptors about the data element ADMISSION_DATE are included in a data dictionary—definition: date patient admitted to the hospital; data type: date; field length: 15; required field: yes; default value: none; template: none. For this data element, data integrity would be better assured if:

    a. The template was defined.

    b. The data type was numeric.

    c. The field was not required.

    d. The field length was longer.

20. In designing an input screen for an EHR, which of the following would be best to capture structured data?

    a. Speech recognition

    b. Drop-down menus

    c. Natural language processing

    d. Document imaging

21. A medical group practice has contracted with an HIM professional to help define the practice's designated record set. Which of the following should the HIM professional perform first to identify the components of the designated record set?

    a. Develop a list of all data elements referencing patients that are included in both paper and electronic systems of the practice.

    b. Develop a list of statutes, regulations, rules, and guidelines that contain requirements affecting the release of health records.

    c. Perform a quality check on all health record systems in the practice.

    d. Develop a listing and categorize all information requests for health information over the past two years.

22. Hospital documentation related to the delivery of patient care such as health records, x-rays, laboratory reports, and consultation reports are owned:

    a. By the hospital

    b. By the patient

    c. By the attending and consulting physician

    d. Jointly by the hospital, physician, and patient

23. Copies of personal health records (PHRs) are considered part of the designated record set when:

    a. Consulted by the provider to gain information on a consumer's health history

    b. Used by the organization to provide treatment

    c. Used by the provider to obtain information on a consumer's prescription history

    d. Used by the organization to determine a consumer's DNR status

24. Which of the following is a true statement about the content of the legal health record?

    a. The legal health record contains only clinical data.

    b. The legal health record may contain metadata.

    c. The legal health record should not include email.

    d. The legal health record should not include diagnostic images.

25. The clinical forms committee is the entity within a healthcare facility that:

    a. Provides oversight for the development, review, and control of forms and computer screens

    b. Is responsible for the EHR implementation and maintenance

    c. Is always a subcommittee of the quality improvement committee

    d. Is an optional function for the HIM department

26. Erin is an HIM professional. She is teaching a class to clinicians about proper documentation in the health record. She should educate the class against doing which of the following?

    a. Obliterating or deleting errors

    b. Leaving existing entries intact

    c. Labeling late entries as being late

    d. Ensuring the legal signature of an individual making a correction accompanies the correction

27. Which of the following is a risk of copy and pasting documentation in the electronic health record?

    a. Reduction in the time required to document

    b. System may not save data

    c. Copying the note in the wrong patient's record

    d. System thinking that the information belongs to the patient from whom the content is being copied

28. Which of the following is the health record component that addresses the patient's current complaints and symptoms and lists that patient's past medical, personal, and family conditions?

    a. Problem list

    b. Medical history

    c. Physical examination

    d. Clinical observation

29. How is the patient registration department assisted by the HIM department?

    a. Assigns the health record number

    b. Processes the healthcare claim

    c. Implements the information systems used by the HIM department

    d. Maintains the information systems used by the HIM department

30. Which of the following is part of qualitative analysis review?

    a. Checking that only approved abbreviations are used

    b. Checking that all forms and reports are present

    c. Checking that documents have patient identification information

    d. Checking that reports requiring authentication have signatures

Domain 2 *Access, Disclosure, Privacy, and Security*

31. Community Hospital is terminating its business associate relationship with a medical transcription company. The transcription company has no further need for any identifiable information that it may have obtained in the course of its business with the hospital. The CFO of the hospital believes that to be HIPAA compliant, all that is necessary is for the termination to be in a formal letter signed by the CEO. In this case, how should the director of HIM advise the CFO?

    a. Determine that a formal letter of termination meets HIPAA requirements and no further action is required.

    b. Confirm that a formal letter of termination meets HIPAA requirements and no further action is required except that the termination notice needs to be retained for seven years.

    c. Confirm that a formal letter of termination is required and that the transcription company must provide the hospital with a certification that all PHI that it had in its possession has been destroyed or returned.

    d. Inform the CFO that business associate agreements cannot be terminated.

32. Which of the following statements is true regarding HIPAA security?

    a. All institutions must implement the same security measures.

    b. Institutions are allowed flexibility in the way they implement HIPAA standards.

    c. All institutions must implement all HIPAA specifications.

    d. A security risk assessment must be performed every year.

33. Access to health records based on protected health information within a healthcare facility should be limited to employees who have a:

    a. Legitimate need for access

    b. Password to access the EHR

    c. Report development program

    d. Signed confidentiality agreement

34. The release of information function requires the HIM professional to have knowledge of:

    a. Clinical coding principles

    b. Database development

    c. Federal and state confidentiality laws

    d. Human resource management

35. When data has been lost in an EHR, which action is taken to remedy this problem?

    a. Build a firewall

    b. Data recovery

    c. Review the audit trail

    d. Develop data integrity plan

36. A tool that identifies when a user logs in and out, what actions he or she takes, and more is called a(n):

    a. Audit trail

    b. Facility access control

    c. Forensic scan

    d. Security management plan

37. A health information technician receives a subpoena *ad testificandum*. To respond to the subpoena, which of the following should the technician do?

    a. Review the subpoena to determine what documents must be produced.

    b. Review the subpoena and notify the hospital administrator.

    c. Review the subpoena and appear at the time and place supplied to give testimony.

    d. Review the subpoena and alert the hospital's risk management department.

38. The admissions director maintains that a notice of privacy practices must be provided to the patient on each admission. How should the HIM director respond?

    a. Notice of privacy practices is required on the first provision of service.

    b. Notice of privacy practices is required every time the patient is provided service.

    c. Notice of privacy practices is only required for inpatient admissions.

    d. Notice of privacy practices is required on the first inpatient admission but for every outpatient encounter.

39. A patient requests copies of her medical records in an electronic format. The hospital does not maintain all the designated record set in an electronic format. How should the hospital respond?

    a. Provide the records in paper format only.

    b. Scan the paper documents so that all records can be sent electronically.

    c. Provide the patient with both paper and electronic copies of the record.

    d. Inform the patient that PHI cannot be sent electronically.

40. On review of the audit trail for an EHR system, the HIM director discovers that a departmental employee who has authorized access to patient records is printing far more records than the average user. In this case, what should the supervisor do?

    a. Reprimand the employee.

    b. Terminate the employee.

    c. Determine what information was printed and why.

    d. Revoke the employee's access privileges.

41. Which of the following definitions best describes the concept of confidentiality?

    a. The expectation that personal information shared by an individual with a healthcare provider during the individual's care will be used only for its intended purpose

    b. The protection of healthcare information from damage, loss, and unauthorized alteration

    c. The right of individuals to control access to their personal health information

    d. The expectation that only individuals with the appropriate authority will be allowed to access healthcare information

42. Ted and Mary are the adoptive parents of Susan, a minor. What is the best way for them to obtain a copy of Susan's operative report?

    a. Wait until Susan is 18 years old.

    b. Present an authorization signed by the court that granted the adoption.

    c. Present an authorization signed by Susan's natural (birth) parents.

    d. Present an authorization that at least one of them (Ted or Mary) has signed.

43. Which of the following individuals may authorize release of health information?

    a. An 86-year-old patient with a diagnosis of advanced dementia

    b. A married 15-year-old father

    c. A 15-year-old minor

    d. The parents of an 18-year-old student

44. A patient requests a copy of his health records. When the request is received, the HIM clerk finds that the records are stored off-site. Which is the longest timeframe the hospital can take to remain in compliance with HIPAA regulations?

    a. Provide copies of the records within 15 days.

    b. Provide copies of the records within 30 days.

    c. Provide copies of the records within 45 days.

    d. Provide copies of the records within 60 days.

45. The right of an individual to keep personal health information from being disclosed to anyone is a definition of:

    a. Confidentiality

    b. Integrity

    c. Privacy

    d. Security

46. What types of covered entity health records are subject to the HIPAA privacy regulations?

    a. Health records in any format

    b. Only health records in electronic format

    c. Only health records from hospitals

    d. Only health records in paper format

47. Typically, the record custodian can testify about which of the following when a party in a legal proceeding is attempting to admit a health record as evidence?

   a. Identification of the record as the one subpoenaed

   b. The care provided to the patient

   c. The qualifications of the treating physician

   d. Identification of the standard of care used to treat the patient

48. The Medical Record Committee is reviewing the privacy policies for a large outpatient clinic. One of the members of the committee remarks that he feels the clinic's practice of calling out a patient's full name in the waiting room is not in compliance with HIPAA regulations and that only the patient's first name should be used. Other committee members disagree with this assessment. What should the HIM director advise the committee?

   a. HIPAA does not allow a patient's name to be announced in a waiting room.

   b. There is no violation of HIPAA in announcing a patient's name, but the committee may want to consider implementing a change that might reduce this practice.

   c. HIPAA allows only the use of the patient's first name.

   d. HIPAA requires that patients be given numbers and only the number be announced.

49. An employee accesses PHI on a computer system that does not relate to her job functions. What security mechanism should have been implemented to minimize this security breach?

   a. Access controls

   b. Audit controls

   c. Contingency controls

   d. Security incident controls

50. Which of the following is true about health information retention?

   a. Retention depends only on accreditation requirements.

   b. Retention periods differ among healthcare facilities.

   c. The operational needs of a healthcare facility cannot be considered.

   d. Retention periods are frequently shorter for health information about minors.

51. Sally has requested an accounting of PHI disclosures from Community Hospital. Which of the following must be included in an accounting of disclosures to comply with this request?

   a. PHI related to treatment, payment, and operations

   b. PHI provided to meet national security or intelligence requirements

   c. PHI sent to a physician who has not treated Sally

   d. PHI released to Sally's attorney upon her request

52. Which of the following is an example of a physical safeguard that should be provided for in a data security program?

   a. Using password protection

   b. Prohibiting the sharing of passwords

   c. Locking computer rooms

   d. Annual employee training

53. An external security threat can be caused by which of the following?

    a. Employees who steal data during work hours

    b. A facility's water pipes bursting

    c. Tornadoes

    d. The failure of a facility's software

54. Which of the following is true regarding the development of health record destruction policies?

    a. All applicable laws must be considered.

    b. The organization must find a way not to destroy any health records.

    c. Health records involved in pending or ongoing litigation may be destroyed.

    d. Only state laws must be considered.

55. As part of your job responsibilities, you are responsible for reviewing audit trails of access to patient information. Which of following activities would you *not* monitor?

    a. Every access to every data element or document type

    b. Whether the person viewed, created, updated, or deleted the information

    c. Physical location on the network where the access occurred

    d. Whether the patient setup an account in the patient portal

56. An employee views a patient's electronic health record. It is a trigger event if:

    a. The employee and patient have the same last name.

    b. The patient was admitted through the emergency department.

    c. The patient is over 89 years old.

    d. A dietitian views a patient's nutrition care plan.

Domain 3 | *Data Analytics and Use*

57. Based on the payment percentages provided in this table, which payer contributes most to the hospital's overall payments?

Payer	Charges	Payments	Adjustment	Charges	Payments	Adjustments
BC/BS	$450,000	$360,000	$90,000	23%	31%	12%
Commercial	$250,000	$200,000	$50,000	13%	17%	6%
Medicaid	$350,000	$75,000	$275,000	18%	6%	36%
Medicare	$750,000	$495,000	$255,000	39%	42%	33%
TRICARE	$150,000	$50,000	$100,000	7%	4%	13%
Total	$1,950,000	$1,180,000	$770,000	100%	100%	100%

    a. BC/BS

    b. Commercial

    c. TRICARE

    d. Medicare

58. Data elements collected on large populations of individuals and stored in databases are referred to as:

    a. Statistics

    b. Information

    c. Aggregate data

    d. Standard

59. Community Hospital wants to compare its hospital-acquired urinary tract infection (UTI) rate for Medicare patients with the national average. The hospital is using the MEDPAR database for its comparison. The MEDPAR database contains 13,000,000 discharges. Of these individuals, 200,000 were admitted with a principal diagnosis of UTI; another 300,000 were admitted with a principal diagnosis of infectious disease, and 700,000 had a diagnosis of hypertension. Given this information, which of the following would provide the best comparison data for Community Hospital?

    a. All individuals in the MEDPAR database

    b. All individuals in the MEDPAR database except those admitted with a principal diagnosis of UTI

    c. All individuals in the MEDPAR database except those admitted with a principal diagnosis of UTI or infectious disease

    d. All individuals in the MEDPAR database except those admitted with a diagnosis of hypertension

60. Given the numbers 47, 20, 11, 33, 30, 30, 35, and 50, what is the median?

    a. 30

    b. 31.5

    c. 32

    d. 35

61. What formatting problem is found in the following table?

Community Hospital Admissions by Gender, 20XX		
Male	3,546	42.4
Female	4,825	57.6
Total	8,371	100

    a. Column headings are missing

    b. Title of the table is missing

    c. Column totals are inaccurate

    d. Variable names are missing

62. Community Hospital had 250 patients in the hospital at midnight on May 1. The hospital admitted 30 patients on May 2. The hospital discharged 40 patients, including deaths, on May 2. Two patients were both admitted and discharged on May 2. What was the total number of inpatient service days for May 2?

    a. 240

    b. 242

    c. 280

    d. 320

63. Community Hospital's HIM department conducted a random sample of 200 inpatient health records to determine the timeliness of the history and physicals completion. Nine records were found to be out of compliance with the 24-hour requirement. Which of the following percentages represents the H&P timeliness rate at Community Hospital?

    a. 4.5%

    b. 21.2%

    c. 66.7%

    d. 95.5%

64. To use a data element for aggregation and reporting, that data element must be:

    a. Abstracted or indexed

    b. Searched

    c. Subject to case finding

    d. Registered

65. Which of the following best represents the definition of the term *data*?

    a. Patient's laboratory value is 50.

    b. Patient's SGOT is higher than 50 and outside of normal limits.

    c. Patient's resting heartbeat is 70, which is within normal range.

    d. Patient's laboratory value is consistent with liver disease.

66. Patient care managers analyze the data documented in the health record to:

    a. Determine the extent and effects of occupational hazards.

    b. Evaluate patterns and trends of patient care.

    c. Generate patient bills and third-party payer claims for reimbursement.

    d. Provide direct patient care.

67. A quality goal for the hospital is that 98 percent of the heart attack patients receive aspirin within 24 hours of arrival at the hospital. In conducting an audit of heart attack patients, the data showed that 94 percent of the patients received aspirin within 24 hours of arriving at the hospital. Given this data, which of the following actions would be best?

    a. Alert the Joint Commission that the hospital has not met its quality goal.

    b. Determine whether there was a medical or other reason why patients were not given aspirin.

    c. Institute an in-service training program for clinical staff on the importance of administering aspirin within 24 hours.

    d. Determine which physicians did not order aspirin.

68. The hospital's Performance Improvement Council has compiled the following data on the volume of procedures performed. Given this data, which procedures should the council scrutinize in evaluating performance?

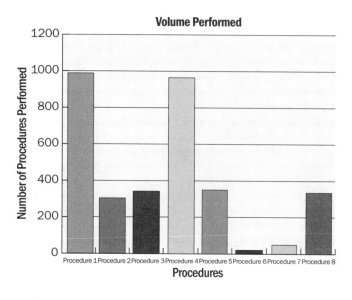

a. Procedures 1, 4

b. Procedures 2, 3, 5

c. Procedures 6, 7

d. Procedures 1, 4, 6, 7

69. A coding supervisor wants to use a fixed percentage random sample of work output to determine coding quality for each coding professional. Given the work output for each of the four coding professionals shown here, how many total records will be needed for the audit if a 5 percent random sample is used?

Fixed Percentage Random Sample Audit Example		
Coding Professional	Work Output	Records for 5% Audit
A	500	
B	480	
C	300	
D	360	

a. 82

b. 156

c. 820

d. 1,550

70. Which tool is used to display performance data over time?

a. Status process control chart

b. Run chart

c. Benchmark

d. Time ladder

71. What is data called that consists of factual details aggregated or summarized from a group of health records that provide no means to identify specific patients?

    a. Original

    b. Source

    c. Protected

    d. Derived

72. Which of the following is an example of how an internal user utilizes secondary data?

    a. State infectious disease reporting

    b. Birth certificates

    c. Death certificates

    d. Benchmarking with other facilities

73. After the types of cases to be included in a cancer registry have been determined, what is the next step in data acquisition?

    a. Case registration

    b. Case definition

    c. Case abstracting

    d. Case finding

74. For research purposes, an advantage of the Healthcare Cost and Utilization Project (HCUP) is that it:

    a. Contains only Medicare data

    b. Is used to determine pay for performance

    c. Contains data on all payer types

    d. Contains bibliographic listings from medical journals

75. Which of the following is true regarding the reporting of communicable diseases?

    a. They must be reported by the patient to the health department.

    b. The diseases to be reported are established by state law.

    c. The diseases to be reported are established by HIPAA.

    d. They are never reported because it would violate the patient's privacy.

76. Based on this output table, what is the average coding test score for the beginner coding professional?

Coding Test Score			
Coding Professional Status	**Mean**	**N**	**Standard Deviation**
Advanced	93.0000	3	5.00000
Intermediate	89.5000	2	0.70711
Beginner	73.3333	3	6.42910
Total	84.7500	8	10.51190

    a. 6.4

    b. 73

    c. 90

    d. 93

77. The HIM manager is analyzing impact to the organization and documenting variations between the current year's diagnosis codes and the proposed new codes for the next fiscal year. This process creates a:

    a. Data chargemaster report

    b. Data dictionary

    c. Database management system

    d. Data map

78. Which of the following is the first step in analyzing data?

    a. Knowing your objectives or purpose of the data analysis

    b. Starting with basic types of data analysis and working up to more sophisticated analysis

    c. Utilizing a statistician to analyze the data

    d. Presenting your findings to administration

79. Sometimes data do not follow a normal distribution and are pulled toward the tails of the curve. When this occurs, it is referred to as having a skewed distribution. Because the mean is sensitive to extreme values or outliers, it gravitates in the direction of the extreme values thus making a long tail when a distribution is skewed. When the tail is pulled toward the right side, it is called a:

    a. Negatively skewed distribution

    b. Positively skewed distribution

    c. Bimodal distribution

    d. Normal distribution

80. In order to better prepare for hurricane season, Seaside Hospital uses a variety of statistical models to help determine how to streamline the admissions process for emergency patients, determine what type of backup generators would meet their needs during a blackout, and determine which additional clinical staff would be needed during future disasters. This type of analytics is referred to as:

    a. Simplistic

    b. Descriptive

    c. Predictive

    d. Prescriptive

81. In order to help the laboratory director understand how this new lab test process fits into the EHR, Dana develops a data flow diagram to show how the information on the new lab test works in the HIS. Dana is performing what type of metadata process?

    a. Descriptive metadata

    b. Structural metadata

    c. Administrative metadata

    d. Prescriptive metadata

Domain 4   *Revenue Cycle Management*

82. A patient presents to Midtown Hospital to have routine lab work completed as part of the monitoring of their diabetes. The patient has recently started a new job and consequently their insurance coverage has changed. The patient was not asked to provide their insurance card, or asked if there had been a change to their insurance coverage since their last visit. Because of the incorrect insurance information listed in the health information system, the claim for this encounter was denied. What revenue cycle front-end process should have addressed the change in the insurance coverage?

    a. Patient assessment

    b. Claims reconciliation

    c. Accounts receivable

    d. Patient registration

83. The discharged, not filed billed report is a daily report used to track accounts that are:

    a. Awaiting payment in accounts receivable

    b. Paid at different rates

    c. In bill hold or in error and awaiting billing

    d. Pulled for quality review

84. Which of the following is a function of the outpatient code editor?

    a. Validate the patient's gender with the procedure codes

    b. Validate the patient's encounter number

    c. Identify unbundling of codes

    d. Identify cases that do not meet medical necessity

85. A patient is admitted for the treatment of dehydration secondary to chemotherapy for primary liver cancer. Intravenous (IV) fluids were administered to the patient. Which of the following should be sequenced as the principal diagnosis?

    a. Dehydration

    b. Chemotherapy

    c. Liver carcinoma

    d. Complication of chemotherapy

86. The first step in an inpatient record review is to verify correct assignment of the:

    a. Record sample

    b. Coding procedures

    c. Principal diagnosis

    d. MS-DRG

87. A patient was seen in the emergency department for chest pain. It was suspected that the patient may have gastroesophageal reflux disease (GERD). The final diagnosis was "Rule out GERD." The correct ICD-10-CM diagnosis code is:

a. K21.9, Gastro-esophageal reflux disease without esophagitis

b. R07.9, Chest pain, unspecified

c. R10.11, Right upper quadrant pain

d. Z03.89, Encounter for observation for other suspected diseases and conditions ruled out

88. A patient received a complete replacement of tunneled centrally inserted central venous catheter with subcutaneous port; replacement performed through original access site (45-year-old patient). Which of the following CPT codes would be most appropriate?

36578	Replacement, catheter only, of central venous access device, with subcutaneous port or pump, central or peripheral insertion site
36580	Replacement, complete, on a non-tunneled centrally inserted central venous catheter, without subcutaneous port or pump, through same venous access
36582	Replacement, complete, of a tunneled centrally inserted central venous access device, with subcutaneous port, through same venous access
36597	Repositioning of previous placed central venous catheter under fluoroscopic guidance

a. 36578

b. 36580

c. 36582, 36597

d. 36582

89. A laparoscopic tubal ligation is undertaken. Which of the following is the correct CPT code assignment?

49320	Laparoscopy, abdomen, peritoneum, and omentum, diagnostic, with or without collection of specimen(s) by brushing or washing (separate procedure)
58662	Laparoscopy, surgical; with fulguration or excision of lesions of the ovary, pelvic viscera, or peritoneal surface by any method
58670	Laparoscopy, surgical; with fulguration of oviducts (with or without transection)
58671	Laparoscopy, surgical; with occlusion of oviducts by device (e.g., band, clip, or Falope ring)

a. 49320, 58662

b. 58670

c. 58671

d. 49320

90. When coding a benign neoplasm of skin of the left upper eyelid, which of the following codes should be used?

> **D23 Other benign neoplasms of skin**
> **Includes:**   benign neoplasm of hair follicles
>   benign neoplasm of sebaceous glands
>   benign neoplasm of sweat glands
>
> **Excludes1:** *benign lipomatous neoplasm of skin (D17.0–D17.3)*
> **Excludes2:** *melanocytic nevi (D22.-)*
>
> **D23.0 Other benign neoplasm of skin of lip**
>   **Excludes1:** *benign neoplasm of vermilion border of lip (D10.0)*
>
> **D23.1 Other benign neoplasm of skin of eyelid, including canthus**
>   **D23.10 Other benign neoplasm of skin of unspecified eyelid, including canthus**
>   **D23.11 Other benign neoplasm of skin of right eyelid, including canthus**
>   D23.111 Other benign neoplasm of skin of right upper eyelid, including canthus
>   D23.112 Other benign neoplasm of skin of right lower eyelid, including canthus
>   **D23.12 Other benign neoplasm of skin of left eyelid, including canthus**
>   D23.121 Other benign neoplasm of skin of left upper eyelid, including canthus
>   D23.122 Other benign neoplasm of skin of left lower eyelid, including canthus
>
> **D23.2 Other benign neoplasm of skin of ear and external auricular canal**
>   **D23.20 Other benign neoplasm of skin of unspecified ear and external auricular canal**
>   **D23.21 Other benign neoplasm of skin of right ear and external auricular canal**
>   **D23.22 Other benign neoplasm of skin of left ear and external auricular canal**

   a. D23.12

   b. D17.0

   c. D23.121

   d. D23.122

91. In CPT, if a patient has two lacerations of the arm that are repaired with simple closures, which of the following would apply for correct coding?

   a. Two CPT codes, one for each laceration

   b. One CPT code for the largest laceration

   c. One CPT code for the most complex closure

   d. One CPT code, adding the lengths of the lacerations together

92. Carolyn works as an inpatient coding professional in a hospital HIM department. She views a lab report in a patient's health record that is positive for staph infection. However, there is no mention of staph in the physician's documentation. What should Carolyn do?

   a. Assign a code for the staph infection.

   b. Put a note in the chart.

   c. Query the physician.

   d. Tell her supervisor.

93. What factor is medical necessity based on?

   a. The beneficial effects of a service for the patient's physical needs and quality of life

   b. The cost of a service compared with the beneficial effects on the patient's health

   c. The availability of a service at the facility

   d. The reimbursement available for a given service

94. A skin lesion was removed from a patient's cheek in the dermatologist's office. The dermatologist documents skin lesion, probable basal cell carcinoma. Which of the following actions should the coding professional take to code this encounter?

    a. Code skin lesion.

    b. Code benign skin lesion.

    c. Code basal cell carcinoma.

    d. Query the dermatologist.

95. A patient had a placenta previa with delivery of twins. The patient had two prior cesarean sections. This was an emergency C-section due to hemorrhage. The appropriate principal diagnosis would be:

    a. Normal delivery

    b. Placenta previa

    c. Twin gestation

    d. Vaginal hemorrhage

96. An alternative to the retrospective coding model is the _____ coding model in which records are coded while the patient is still an inpatient.

    a. Concurrent

    b. Analytical

    c. Prospective

    d. Auxiliary

97. The facility's Medicare case-mix index has dropped, although other statistical measures appear constant. The CFO suspects coding errors. What type of coding quality review should be performed?

    a. Random audit

    b. Focused audit

    c. Compliance audit

    d. External audit

98. A patient was admitted to the hospital with symptoms of a stroke and secondary diagnoses of COPD and hypertension. The patient was subsequently discharged from the hospital with a principal diagnosis of cerebral vascular accident and secondary diagnoses of catheter-associated urinary tract infection, COPD, and hypertension. Which of the following diagnoses would be reported as present on admission (POA)?

    a. Catheter-associated urinary tract infection, COPD, Hypertension

    b. Cerebral vascular accident, COPD, Catheter-associated urinary tract infection

    c. Cerebral vascular accident, COPD, Hypertension

    d. Hypertension, Catheter-associated urinary tract infection, Cerebral vascular accident

99. A Staghorn calculus of the left renal pelvis was treated earlier in the week by lithotripsy and is now removed via a percutaneous nephrostomy tube. What is the root operation performed for this procedure?

   a. Destruction

   b. Extirpation

   c. Extraction

   d. Fragmentation

100. A patient has a malunion of an intertrochanteric fracture of the right hip, which is treated with a proximal femoral osteotomy by incision. What is the correct ICD-10-PCS code for this procedure?

Section	Body System	Root Operation	Body Part	Approach	Device	Qualifier
Medical and Surgical	Lower Bones	Excision	Upper Femur, Right	Open	No Device	No Qualifier
0	Q	B	6	0	Z	Z

Section	Body System	Root Operation	Body Part	Approach	Device	Qualifier
Medical and Surgical	Lower Bones	Division	Upper Femur, Right	Open	No Device	No Qualifier
0	Q	8	6	0	Z	Z

Section	Body System	Root Operation	Body Part	Approach	Device	Qualifier
Medical and Surgical	Lower Joints	Excision	Hip Joint, Right	Open	No Device	No Qualifier
0	S	B	9	0	Z	Z

Section	Body System	Root Operation	Body Part	Approach	Device	Qualifier
Medical and Surgical	Lower Joints	Release	Hip Joint, Right	Open	No Device	No Qualifier
0	S	N	9	0	Z	Z

   a. 0QB60ZZ

   b. 0Q860ZZ

   c. 0SB90ZZ

   d. 0SN90ZZ

101. Local coverage determinations (LCD) describe when and under what circumstances which of the following is met:

   a. MACs

   b. Medical necessity

   c. NCDs

   d. Proper administration of benefits

102. The practice of undercoding can affect a hospital's MS-DRG case mix in which of the following ways?

    a. Makes it lower than warranted by the actual service and resource intensity of the facility

    b. Makes it higher than warranted by the actual service and resource intensity of the facility

    c. Hospital's MS-DRG case mix is never monitored so there is no impact

    d. Coding has nothing to do with a hospital's MS-DRG case mix

103. If a physician does not provide a diagnosis to justify the medical necessity of a service, the provider may obtain payment from the patient:

    a. For the balance due after Medicare has paid

    b. Only if both Medicare and any supplemental insurance have been billed and settled

    c. Never—providers may not bill Medicare patients for amounts unpaid by Medicare

    d. Only if a properly executed ABN was obtained before the service was provided

104. The utilization manager's role is essential to:

    a. Analyze the estimate of benefits (EOBs) received

    b. Capture all relevant charges for the patient's account

    c. Prevent denials for inappropriate levels of service

    d. Verify the patient has insurance

105. Clinical documentation improvement (CDI) programs use metrics to evaluate the effectiveness of their program. Which of the following is the most widely used key indicator for a CDI program?

    a. Case-mix index

    b. Severity of illness score

    c. Accounts receivable index

    d. Risk mortality score

106. From the information provided in the following table, what percentage will the facility be paid for procedure 25500?

Billing Number	Status Indicator	CPT/HCPCS	APC
998323	V	99285–25	0612
998323	T	25500	0044
998323	X	72050	0261
998323	S	72128	0283
998323	S	70450	0283

    a. 0%

    b. 50%

    c. 75%

    d. 100%

107. Joe Carlson was admitted to Community Hospital. Two days later, he was transferred to Big Medical Center for further evaluation and treatment. He was discharged to home after three days with a qualified transfer DRG from Big Medical Center. Community Hospital will receive from Medicare:

    a. The full DRG amount, and Big Medical Center will receive a per diem rate for the three-day stay

    b. A per diem rate for the two-day stay, and Big Medical Center will receive the full DRG payment

    c. The full DRG amount, and Big Medical Center will bill Community Hospital a per diem rate for the three-day stay

    d. No payment; Community Hospital must bill Big Medical Center a per diem rate for the two-day stay

108. Quality Improvement Organizations perform medical peer review of Medicare and Medicaid claims through a review of which of the following?

    a. Validity of hospital diagnosis and procedure coding data completeness

    b. Appropriateness of EHR used

    c. Policies, procedures, and standards of conduct

    d. Professional standards

109. The accounting for all reportable services and supplies rendered to a patient is called:

    a. Department code

    b. Revenue code

    c. Charge capture

    d. Prior authorization

110. John was in a motor vehicle accident and brought to the emergency department at the local hospital. He presented with a severe headache, and pain and abrasions on both forearms due to airbag deployment. The patient was taken for x-rays of the forearms and a CT scan of the head. The provider documented contusions and abrasions of both forearms and headache, as no significant findings were found on the radiology procedures. The coding manager was reviewing claims denials and found that John's insurance had denied the claim for the CT of the head. Upon further review, the coding manager discovered that the coding professional neglected to code the headache diagnosis. Which of the following actions should be taken to manage this denial?

    a. No action should be taken as the insurance should not pay for the CT scan.

    b. The coding professional should add the diagnosis of headache and the claim should be resubmitted.

    c. The coding professional should add the diagnosis of abnormal findings, radiologic exam and the claim should be resubmitted.

    d. No action should be taken as the claim cannot be resubmitted to the insurance company.

111. Which of the following is a service common for hospitals and large physician practices to provide to their patients as they try to manage payment for services? This service can be in the form of offering payment plans, healthcare loans, or payment support from manufacturers of high-cost pharmaceuticals.

    a. Patient financial counseling

    b. Patient portal access

    c. Balance billing

    d. Explanation of benefits

112. The determination of the reimbursement amount based on the beneficiary's insurance plan benefits is called:

    a. Charge capture

    b. Adjudication

    c. Adjustment

    d. Revenue management

113. Which of the following statements is true about including modifiers in the charge description master (CDM)?

    a. Modifiers should be widely used in the CDM because they do not impact reimbursement.

    b. Modifiers should be widely used in the CDM because they do not change the meaning of the HCPCS code they are attached to.

    c. Modifiers should be used sparingly in the CDM because documentation in the medical record must support the application of the modifier.

    d. Modifiers should never be used in the CDM because it is against the rules.

Domain 5 *Compliance*

114. The leaders of a healthcare organization are expected to select an organization-wide performance improvement approach and to clearly define how all levels of the organization will monitor and address improvement issues. The Joint Commission requires ongoing data collection that might require improvement for which of the following areas?

    a. Operative and other invasive procedures, medication management, and blood and blood product use

    b. Blood and blood product use, medication management, and appointment to the board of directors

    c. Medication management, marketing strategy, and blood use

    d. Operative and other invasive procedures, appointments to the board of directors, and restraint and seclusion use

115. In developing an internal audit review program, which of the following would be risk areas that should be targeted for audit?

    a. Admission diagnosis and complaints

    b. Chargemaster description

    c. Clinical laboratory results

    d. Radiology orders

116. Which of the following practices is an appropriate coding compliance activity?

    a. Reviewing all accurately paid claims

    b. Developing procedures for identifying coding errors

    c. Providing a financial incentive for coding claims improperly

    d. Instructing coding professionals to code diagnoses and submit the bill before all applicable information is documented in the health record

117. The goal of coding compliance programs is to prevent:

    a. Accusations of fraud and abuse

    b. Delays in claims processing

    c. Billing errors

    d. Inaccurate code assignments

118. A coding professional's misrepresentation of the patient's clinical picture through intentional incorrect coding or the omission of diagnosis or procedure codes would be an example of:

    a. Healthcare fraud

    b. Payment optimization

    c. Payment reduction

    d. Healthcare creativity

119. When performing a coding audit, a health record technician discovers that an inpatient coding professional is assigning diagnosis and procedure codes specifically for the purpose of obtaining a higher level of reimbursement. The coding professional believes that this practice helps the hospital increase its revenue. Which of the following should be done in this case?

    a. Compliment the coding professional for taking initiative in helping the hospital.

    b. Report the coding professional to the FBI for coding fraud.

    c. Counsel the coding professional and stop the practice immediately.

    d. Provide the coding professional with incentive pay for her actions.

120. The risk manager's principal tool for capturing the facts about potentially compensable events is the:

    a. Accident report

    b. RM report

    c. Occurrence report

    d. Event report

121. A hospital receives a valid request from a patient for copies of her health records. The HIM clerk who is preparing the records removes copies of the patient's records from another hospital where the patient was previously treated. According to HIPAA regulations, was this action correct?

    a. No; the records from the previous hospital are considered to be included in the designated record set and should be given to the patient.

    b. Yes; this is hospital policy for which HIPAA has no control.

    c. No; the records from the previous hospital are not included in the designated record set but should be released anyway.

    d. Yes; HIPAA only requires that current records be produced for the patient.

122. The deception or misrepresentation by a healthcare provider that may result in a false or fictitious claim for inappropriate payment by Medicare or other insurers for items or services either not rendered or rendered to a lesser extent than described in the claim is:

    a. Healthcare fraud

    b. Optimization

    c. Upcoding

    d. Healthcare abuse

123. What should be done when the HIM department's chart analysis error rate is too high, or its accuracy rate is too low based on policy?

    a. Re-audit the problem area

    b. The problem should be treated as an isolated incident

    c. The formula for determining the rate may need to be adjusted

    d. Corrective action should be taken to meet the department standards

124. The Department of Health and Human Services has identified that Community Hospital is guilty of fraud. It was determined that the facility tried to comply with standards, but their efforts failed. What category of fraud and abuse prevention does this fall into?

    a. Reasonable cause

    b. Reasonable diligence

    c. Willful neglect

    d. Willful defiance

125. City Hospital submitted 175 claims where they unbundled laboratory charges. They were overpaid by $75 on each claim. What is the fine for City Hospital if triple damages are applied?

    a. $40,300

    b. $39,375

    c. $26,250

    d. $13,125

126. What resource should the facility compliance officer consult to provide information on new and ongoing reviews or audits each year in programs administered by the Department of Health and Human Services?

    a. Regional health information organizations

    b. Corporate compliance plans

    c. OIG website

    d. *Federal Register*

127. When a staff member documents in the health record that an incident report was completed about a specific incident, in a legal proceeding how is the confidentiality of the incident report affected?

    a. There is no impact.

    b. The person making the entry in the health record may not be called as a witness in trial.

    c. The incident report likely becomes discoverable because it is mentioned in a discoverable document.

    d. The incident report cannot be discovered even though it is mentioned in a discoverable document.

128. The basic functions of healthcare risk management programs are similar for most organizations and should include which of the following?

    a. Reporting of claims, initiating an investigation of claims, protecting the primary and secondary health records, negotiating settlements, managing litigations, and using information for claim's resolution in performance management activities

    b. Risk acceptance, risk avoidance, risk reduction or minimization, and risk transfer

    c. Safety management, security management, claims management, technology management, and facilities management

    d. Risk identification and analysis, loss prevention and reduction, and claims management

129. A provider's office calls to retrieve emergency room records for a patient's follow-up appointment. The HIM professional refused to release the emergency department records without a written authorization from the patient. Was this action in compliance?

    a. No; the records are needed for continued care of the patient, so no authorization is required.

    b. Yes; the release of all records requires written authorization from the patient.

    c. No; permission of the ER physician was not obtained.

    d. Yes; one covered entity cannot request the records from another covered entity.

130. The HIM improvement team wants to identify the causes of poor documentation compliance in the health record. Which of the following tools would best aid the team in identifying the root cause of the problem?

    a. Flowchart

    b. Fishbone diagram

    c. Pareto chart

    d. Scatter diagram

131. Which of the following has created ethical issues based on security, interoperability, and record integrity?

    a. Accreditation processes

    b. Telemedicine

    c. Sensitive data

    d. Electronic health record

132. The HIM manager is reviewing the performance metrics for her department and notices that the ROI staff is taking over five days to fulfill a request for PHI. The standard for the ROI staff to complete this task is three days. What metric is the HIM manager monitoring for department compliance?

    a. ROI request sources

    b. ROI staffing

    c. ROI productivity

    d. ROI turnaround time

133. In order to provide ongoing compliance education to the coding staff, the coding manager regularly reviews these policies for information regarding reasonable and necessary provisions for a supply, procedure, or service. The policies include a list of codes describing which conditions are a medical necessity and which conditions do not warrant medical necessity. What policies is the coding manager reviewing?

    a. Value-based purchasing

    b. Local coverage determinations

    c. Clinical documentation integrity

    d. Price transparency

Domain 6   *Leadership*

134. Based on a productivity log, a coding professional completed 23 charts during a 7.5-hour workday. The performance standard is four charts per hour. How many charts did he code per hour? Round to the nearest whole number.

    a. 2

    b. 3

    c. 4

    d. 23

135. An HIM department is projecting workforce needs for its document scanning process. The intent of the department is to scan patient records at the time of discharge, providing a 24-hour turnaround time. The hospital has an average daily discharge of 120 patients, and each patient record has an average of 200 pages. Given the benchmarks listed here, what is the least amount of work hours needed each day to meet a 24-hour turnaround time?

National Benchmarks for Document Scanning Processes	
Function	**Expectations per Worked Hour**
Prepping	340–500 images
Scanning	1,200–2,400 images
Quality Control	1,600–2,000 images
Indexing	600–800 images

    a. 100 hours

    b. 146 hours

    c. 1,000 hours

    d. 3,740 hours

136. The HIM department is developing a system to track coding productivity. The director wants the system to track the productivity of each coding professional by productive hours worked per day, health record ID, and type of records coded; as well as provide weekly productivity reports and analyses. Which of the following tools would be best to use for this purpose?

    a. Word-processing documents

    b. Paper log book

    c. Spreadsheet

    d. Database management system

137. Which phase in the project life cycle is where installation of equipment or construction begins, and any policy or procedure manuals should be prepared for distribution?

    a. Closure

    b. Execution

    c. Initiation

    d. Planning

138. Zachary is the new EHR coordinator. He has written all the EHR training material for employees. During the initial training, he stresses he has worked with various departments to ensure that different systems communicate and exchange information without corrupting the data. The ability of these different information systems and software applications to communicate and exchange data is referred to as:

    a. Interoperability

    b. Certification

    c. NLP

    d. Meaningful Use

139. The HIM and IT departments are working together to justify additional employee password training. The additional training would cost approximately $100,000 with the expectation that password calls to the IT help desk will be reduced by 20 percent. The IT department has done a cost analysis of help desk calls solving password issues. Given this data and approximately 40 password calls per day, can the cost of the additional training be justified?

Costs Associated with Each IT Help Desk Call to Resolve Password Issues	
Personnel	Cost
User's time—30 minutes	$15
Telephone cost—30 minutes	$2
Call Desk time—30 minutes	$16
Call Desk IS facilities time	$17
Total	$50

    a. Training will provide $146,000 savings in help desk support and can be justified.

    b. The results of training will provide $365,000 savings in help desk support and can be justified.

    c. The cost of training will be recouped in less than half a year and can be justified.

    d. The cost of training is not justified because qualitative results cannot be measured to calculate a return on investment.

140. As part of Community Hospital's organization-wide quality improvement initiative, the HIM director is establishing benchmarks for all the divisions within the HIM department. The following table shows sample productivity benchmarks for record analysis the director found through a literature search. Given this information, how should the director proceed in establishing benchmarks for the department?

Sample Productivity Benchmarks			
Productivity Benchmarks	**Per Hour**		
Function	**Low**	**Average**	**High**
Analysis (charts per hour)			
Inpatient		8	20
Observation/outpatient surgery/newborn/maternity	5	14	60
Other outpatient		20	120

a. Determine whether the source of the benchmark data is from a comparable institution.

b. Use the low benchmark example as a beginning point for implementation.

c. Contact the hospital statistician to determine whether the data are relevant.

d. Use the average benchmark example as a beginning point for implementation.

141. An audit of the document imaging process reveals that the HIM department staff is scanning 250 pages per hour and indexing 114 pages per hour. If the department is meeting its performance standard for scanning, but is only meeting 60 percent of the indexing standard, how many more pages per hour must be indexed to meet the indexing standard?

a. 45.6 pages

b. 68.4 pages

c. 76 pages

d. 190 pages

142. The HIM director has put together a group of department employees to develop coding benchmarks for the number and types of charts to be coded per work hour. The group includes seven employees from the analysis, transcription, release of information, and coding sections. No managers are included on the team because the HIM director wants a bottom-up approach to benchmark development. What fundamental team leadership mistake is the HIM director making with composition of the team?

a. Insufficient knowledge of team members

b. Too many team members

c. Unspecific team charge

d. Too few team members

143. Which of the following is a positive aspect of using employee self-appraisal as a source of data for performance appraisal?

a. Employees are in the best position to provide objective review without overstatement.

b. The supervisor is kept informed of the employee's accomplishments.

c. Appraiser and employee training on the purpose and procedures of this process is essential.

d. Peer pressure of evaluation can motivate team members to be more productive.

144. Dr. Wesson is looking for a new EHR system for her practice. Since you are the HIM director, she asks you what is absolutely essential in an EHR system? You tell her EHRs must prove they have been tested to perform up to national standards. Which of the following is used to describe health information technologies that have been tested and certified to perform up to national standards?

    a. CEHRT

    b. CERT

    c. CPOE

    d. ONC

145. One release of information (ROI) specialist handles requests from insurance and managed care companies. Another handles requests from attorneys and courts. Each completes all steps in the business process from beginning to end. This is an example of which of the following?

    a. Serial work division

    b. Job sharing

    c. Job rotation

    d. Parallel work division

146. When reviewing the monthly performance report, a manager noticed the coding accuracy rate was below standard. She considered whether this difference might be related to a recent change in systems or attributed to another factor. This manager is performing which of the following?

    a. Performance measurement

    b. Workforce planning

    c. Work observation study

    d. Variance analysis

147. In designing input by clinicians for an EHR system, which of the following would be effective for a clinician when the data are repetitive and the vocabulary used is fairly limited?

    a. Drop-down menus

    b. Point and click fields

    c. Speech recognition

    d. Structured templates

148. This planning technique provides a structure that requires the project team to identify the order and projected duration of activities needed to complete a project:

    a. Gantt chart

    b. Flowchart

    c. Pie chart

    d. PERT chart

149. Performance monitoring is data driven and the HIM department needs access to data in order to make important decisions. One way to provide real-time data and important information that can be monitored at a glance is to use which of the following?

    a. Benchmark

    b. Dashboards

    c. Pareto chart

    d. Time ladder

150. The RHIT supervisor for the scanning and quality control section of Community Clinic is developing a staffing schedule for the year. The clinic is open 260 days per year and has an average of 500 clinic visits per day. The standard for scanning records is 50 records per hour. The standard for quality control of scanning of records is 40 records per hour. Given these standards, how many productive hours will be required daily to scan and quality control records for each clinic day?

   a. 10 hours per day

   b. 11.11 hours per day

   c. 12.5 hours per day

   d. 22.5 hours per day

PRACTICE EXAM 2

Domain 1 *Data Content, Structure, and Information Governance*

1. Policies and procedures need to be in place to address amendments and corrections in the EHR. In the event an amendment, addendum, or deletion needs to be made, which of the following should occur?

   a. The EHR should retain only the latest version of the document in order to avoid confusion as it is not necessary to document who made a change and when.

   b. The EHR should not allow any amendments, addendums, or deletions of electronic documents as this violates accreditation standards.

   c. The EHR should retain the previous version of the document and identify who made the change along with the date and time that the change was made.

   d. The EHR is not capable of allowing documentation changes. If a document needs to be amended, it must printed, redlined, and scanned into the EHR.

2. Which of the following is a correct statement regarding DNR orders?

   a. A DNR is a form of advance directive and only requires the patient's desire for the withholding of care.

   b. The record should be clearly marked to indicate the presence of a DNR order.

   c. A DNR replaces the need for an advance directive since it is the ultimate in advance directive notifications.

   d. The Patient Self-Determination Act is federal so there are no differences in state law that need to be consulted.

3. Which of the following represents the required documentation elements needed to be included in a patient's health record when a surgical procedure is performed?

   a. Operative report, anesthesia report, recovery room report

   b. Discharge summary, anesthesia report, operative report

   c. Recovery room report, physical therapy notes, operative report

   d. Operative report, discharge summary, anesthesia report

4. Dr. Smith wants to use a lot of free text in his EHR. What should be your response?

   a. Good idea, Dr. Smith. This allows you to customize the documentation for each patient.

   b. Dr. Smith, we recommend that you do not use any free text in the EHR.

   c. Dr. Smith, we recommend that you should use free text only in your more complex cases.

   d. Dr. Smith, we recommend that you use little, if any, free text in the EHR.

5. A hospital's EHR defines the expected values of the gender data element as female, male, and unknown. This type of specificity is known as:

   a. Data precision

   b. Data consistency

   c. Data granularity

   d. Data comprehensiveness

6. Cancer registries are maintained by hospitals:

    a. By federal law or state law

    b. Voluntarily or by state law

    c. Voluntarily or by federal law

    d. By mandate from the American College of Surgeons

7. Which of the following reports includes names of the surgeon and assistants, date, duration, and description of the procedure and any specimens removed?

    a. Anesthesia report

    b. Laboratory report

    c. Operative report

    d. Pathology report

8. Clinical documentation systems that support clinical decision-making capture data via which of the following?

    a. Alerting programs

    b. Digital dictation

    c. Scanned images

    d. Templates

9. In a routine health record quantitative analysis review, it was found that a physician dictated a discharge summary on 1/26/20XX. Because of unexpected complications; however, the patient was discharged two days after the discharge summary was dictated. What would be the best course of action in this case?

    a. Request that the physician dictate an addendum to the discharge summary.

    b. Have the record analyst note the date discrepancy.

    c. Request that the physician dictate another discharge summary.

    d. File the record as complete because the discharge summary includes all the pertinent patient information.

10. Which of the following data sets would be most helpful in developing a hospital trauma data registry?

    a. DEEDS

    b. MDS

    c. OASIS

    d. UACDS

11. Identify the report where the following information would be found: "HEENT: Reveals the tympanic membranes, nares, and pharynx to be clear. No obvious head trauma. CHEST: Good bilateral chest sounds."

    a. Discharge summary

    b. Health history

    c. Medical laboratory report

    d. Physical examination

12. After implementing a new EHR, the HIM department is noticing that documents are occasionally found in the wrong health record or are mislabeled. Which of the following would be the best approach to manage these errors in the EHR?

    a. Ignore them because it does not matter.

    b. Establish an error-management team to receive notice of these instances and correct them.

    c. Establish a policy for HIM staff to be more careful.

    d. Report these issues to the IT department to resolve them.

13. Which of the following would be the best technique to ensure nurses do not omit any essential information on the nursing intake assessment in an EHR?

    a. Add validation edits on all essential fields.

    b. Provide an input mask for essential data fields.

    c. Make all essential data fields required by using a template.

    d. Provide sufficient space for all essential fields.

14. The link that tracks patient, person, or member activity within healthcare organizations and across patient care settings is known as:

    a. Enterprise master patient index (EMPI)

    b. Audit trail

    c. Case-mix management

    d. Electronic document management system (EDMS)

15. Which of the following would be the best technique to ensure that registration clerks consistently use the correct notation for assigning admission date in an EHR?

    a. Make admission date a required field.

    b. Provide a template for entering data in the field.

    c. Make admission date a numeric field.

    d. Provide sufficient space for input of data.

16. Which type of data identifies the patient (such as name, health record number, address, and telephone number)?

    a. Accession data

    b. Indicator data

    c. Reference data

    d. Demographic data

17. Managing an organization's data and those who enter it is an ongoing challenge requiring active administration and oversight. This can be accomplished by the organization through management of which of the following?

    a. Data dictionary

    b. Data warehouse

    c. Data mapping

    d. Data set

18. A coding analyst consistently enters the wrong code for patient gender in the computer billing system. What measures should be in place to minimize this data entry error?

    a. Access controls

    b. Audit trail

    c. Edit checks

    d. Password controls

19. Two coding professionals have found the same abbreviation in two records. One abbreviation of "O.D." was used on an eye health record to mean "right eye." The other abbreviation in another patient's record was used to mean "overdose" in an abuse record. What data quality component is lacking here?

    a. Timeliness

    b. Completeness

    c. Security

    d. Consistency

20. Which of the following is the goal of the quantitative analysis performed by HIM professionals?

    a. Ensuring that the health record is legible

    b. Verifying that health professionals are providing appropriate care

    c. Identifying deficiencies early so they can be corrected

    d. Ensuring bills are correct

21. The credentialing process of independent practitioners within a healthcare organization must be defined in:

    a. Hospital policies and procedures

    b. Medical staff bylaws

    c. Accreditation regulations

    d. Hospital licensure rules

22. Which of the following is true about the legal health record?

    a. It is inadmissible into evidence.

    b. It may not be hybrid.

    c. It must consist in part on paper.

    d. It will be disclosed upon request.

23. Physician orders for DNR should be consistent with:

    a. Patient's advance directive

    b. Patient's bill of rights

    c. Notice of privacy practices

    d. Authorization for release of information

24. Which of the following is an argument against the use of the copy and paste function in the EHR?

    a. Inability to identify the author

    b. Inability to print the data out

    c. The time that it takes to copy and paste the documentation

    d. The users will not know how to perform the copy and paste function

25. Clara maintains and updates an individual health record for herself as a tool she can use to collect, track, and share her past and current information about her health with providers. What is this tool called?

    a. Hybrid health record

    b. Paper health record

    c. Duplicate health record

    d. Personal health record

26. The EHR may have multiple versions of the same document; for example, a signed and unsigned copy. How can a healthcare organization manage version control of documents in the EHR?

    a. Delete old versions and retain only the most recent version.

    b. Employ policies and procedures to control which version(s) is displayed.

    c. Do not consider signed and unsigned documents to be two versions.

    d. Previous versions are accessible to administration only.

27. A patient's gender, phone number, address, next of kin, and insurance policy holder information would be considered what kind of data?

    a. Clinical data

    b. Authorization data

    c. Administrative data

    d. Consent data

28. Which of the following is true about information assets?

    a. Information considered to add value to an organization

    b. Data entered into a patient's health record by a provider

    c. Clearly defined elements required to be documented in the health record

    d. A list of all data elements added within a record

29. Which of the following is *not* a recommended guideline for maintaining integrity in the health record?

    a. Specifying consequences for the falsification of information

    b. Requiring periodic training covering the falsification of information and information security

    c. Ensuring documentation that is being changed is permanently deleted from the record

    d. Prohibiting the entry of false information into any of the organization's records

30. The HIM manager was asked by the medical director to present the hospital's policy on deletion of erroneous information from the electronic health record (EHR) to the medical staff. This policy requires that the original documentation is retained in the EHR along with the corrected documentation. Which of the following is a key component of this policy?

    a. The new documentation must be reviewed by the chief of the medical staff.

    b. Natural language processing would be utilized to delete erroneous information.

    c. The new and old documentation would be included in the same document with a comment section.

    d. The new documentation needs to be reviewed by the risk manager.

Domain 2 | *Access, Disclosure, Privacy, and Security*

31. A dietary department donated its old laptop to a school. Some old patient data were still on the computer. What controls would have minimized this security breach?

    a. Access controls

    b. Device and media controls

    c. Facility access controls

    d. Workstation controls

32. An HIM technician was alerted by registration that the system has a record for John Smith with two different birthdates. After an investigation the technician determined the documentation was for two different patients, both named John Smith, who have the same health record number in the EHR. This is an example of:

    a. Overlap

    b. Overlay

    c. Duplicate

    d. Purge

33. A coding compliance manager is reviewing a tool that identifies when a user logs in and out, what he or she does, and more. What is the manager reviewing?

    a. Audit trail

    b. Facility access control

    c. Forensics

    d. Security management plan

34. Which of the following should be considered first when establishing health record retention policies?

    a. State retention requirements

    b. Accreditation standards

    c. AHIMA's retention guidelines

    d. Federal requirements

35. A hospital is planning to allow coding professionals to work at home. The hospital is in the process of identifying strategies to minimize the security risks associated with this practice. Which of the following would be best to ensure that data breaches are minimized when the home computer is unattended?

    a. Username and password

    b. Encryption

    c. Cable locks

    d. Automatic session log-off

36. Recently, a local professional athlete was admitted to your facility for a procedure. During this patient's hospital stay, access logs may need to be checked daily in order to determine:

    a. Whether access by employees is appropriate

    b. If the patient is satisfied with their stay

    c. If it is necessary to order prescriptions for the patient

    d. Whether the care to the patient meets quality standards

37. Community Hospital's physicians have requested the ability to access the EHR from their offices and from home. What advice should the HIM director provide?

    a. HIPAA regulations do not allow this type of access.

    b. This access would be covered under the release of PHI for treatment purposes and poses no security or confidentiality threats.

    c. Access can be permitted providing that appropriate safeguards are put in place to protect against threats to security.

    d. Access can be permitted because the physicians are on the medical staff of the hospital and are covered by HIPAA as employees.

38. What is the term used most often to describe the individual within an organization who is responsible for protecting health information in conjunction with the court system?

    a. Administrator of records

    b. Custodian of records

    c. Director of records

    d. Supervisor of records

39. A hospital HIM department receives a subpoena *duces tecum* for records of a former patient. When the health record technician goes to retrieve the patient's health records, it is discovered that the records being subpoenaed have been purged in accordance with the state retention laws. In this situation, how should the HIM department respond to the subpoena?

    a. Submit a certification of destruction in response to the subpoena.

    b. Inform defense and plaintiff lawyers that the records no longer exist.

    c. Refuse the subpoena since no records exist.

    d. Contact the clerk of the court and explain the situation.

40. A home health agency has a computer system where its nurses document home care services on a laptop computer taken to the patient's home. The laptops will connect to the agency's computer network. The agency is in the process of identifying strategies to minimize the risks associated with the practice. Which of the following would be the best practice to protect laptop and network data from a virus introduced from an external device?

    a. Biometrics

    b. Encryption

    c. Personal firewall software

    d. Session terminations

41. A subpoena *duces tecum* compels the recipient to:

    a. Serve on a jury

    b. Answer a complaint

    c. Testify at trial

    d. Bring records to a legal proceeding

42. Which of the following situations is considered a breach of PHI?

    a. A nurse views the record of a patient that she is not caring for.

    b. A patient's attorney is sent records not authorized by that patient.

    c. A nurse starts to place PHI in a public area where a patient is standing and immediately picks it up.

    d. An HIM employee keys in the incorrect health record number but closes it out as soon as it is realized.

43. Which of the following principles is being followed when a health information management professional ensures that patient information is only released to those who have a legal right to access it?

    a. Autonomy

    b. Beneficence

    c. Justice

    d. Nonmaleficence

44. An individual's right to control access to his or her personal information is known as:

    a. Security

    b. Confidentiality

    c. Privacy

    d. Access control

45. Community Hospital provides voice recognition services for office notes of the private patients of physicians. All these physicians have medical staff privileges at the hospital. This is an essential service to the physicians and will provide additional revenue for the hospital. Which of the following should the hospital HIM director advise in order to comply with HIPAA regulations?

    a. Each physician practice should obtain a business associate agreement with the hospital.

    b. The hospital should obtain a business associate agreement with each physician practice.

    c. Because the physicians all have medical staff privileges, no business associate agreement is necessary.

    d. Because the physicians are part of an Organized Health Care Arrangement with the hospital, no business associate agreement is necessary.

46. Community Hospital has a storage facility with older records that must be retained to meet retention laws and guidelines. The HIM professional has been tasked with removing health records from an associated clinic of patients who have not been treated for a specific period of time and sending those records to the storage area. This process is called:

    a. Purging records

    b. Assembling records

    c. Logging records

    d. Cycling records

47. Which of the following refers to guarding against improper information modification or destruction?

    a. Confidentiality

    b. Integrity

    c. Privacy

    d. Security

48. Spoliation can be defined as which of the following?

    a. It is required after a legal hold is imposed.

    b. It is the negligent destruction or changing of information.

    c. It is destroying, changing, or hiding evidence intentionally.

    d. It can only be performed on records that are involved in a court proceeding.

49. Which of the following would be considered a security vulnerability?

    a. Lack of laptop encryption

    b. Workforce employees

    c. Tornado

    d. Electrical outage

50. When an individual requests a copy of the PHI or agrees to accept summary or explanatory information, the covered entity may:

    a. Impose a reasonable cost-based fee

    b. Not charge the individual

    c. Impose any fee authorized by state statute

    d. Charge only for the cost of the paper on which the information is printed

51. Release of birth and death information to public health authorities:

    a. Is prohibited without patient consent

    b. Is prohibited without patient authorization

    c. Is a public health activities disclosure that does not require patient authorization

    d. Requires both patient consent and authorization

52. Which of the following is a characteristic of breach notification?

    a. It is only required when 500 or more individuals are affected.

    b. It applies to both secured and unsecured PHI.

    c. It applies when one person's PHI is breached.

    d. Is only applies when 20 or more individuals are affected.

53. With regard to training in PHI policies and procedures:

    a. Every member of the covered entity's workforce must be trained.

    b. Only individuals employed by the covered entity must be trained.

    c. Training only needs to occur when there are material changes to the policies and procedures.

    d. Documentation of training is not required.

54. Typically, healthcare facilities should retain the master patient index:

    a. For at least 5 years

    b. For at least 10 years

    c. For at least 25 years

    d. Permanently

55. Mary's PHI has been breached. Of which of the following does Mary *not* need to be notified?

    a. Who committed the breach

    b. Date the breach was discovered

    c. Types of unsecured PHI involved

    d. What she may do to protect herself

56. HIPAA requires a covered entity to establish policy to ensure that protected health information cannot identify a specific individual. One method used to meet this deidentification standard is the expert determination model. The expert determination model requires these four steps:

    1. Determine the statistical and scientific method to be used to determine the risk of reidentification.

    2. Analyze and assess the risk to the deidentified data.

    3. The expert applies the method to the deidentified data.

    4. The facility should choose the expert for the deidentification analysis.

    What is the correct order in which these steps should be performed?

    a. 4, 1, 2, 3

    b. 1, 2, 3, 4

    c. 2, 4, 3, 1

    d. 4, 1, 3, 2

Domain 3 Data Analytics and Use

57. A consumer nonprofit organization wants to conduct studies on the quality of care provided to Medicare patients in a specific region. An HIT professional has been hired to manage this project. The nonprofit organization asks the HIT professional about the viability of using billing data as the basis for its analysis. Which of the following would *not* be a quality consideration in using billing data?

    a. Accuracy of the data

    b. Consistency of the data

    c. Appropriateness of the data elements

    d. Cost to process the data

58. The HIM manager recently performed an audit of health record documentation in the EHR looking for reports that had been indexed incorrectly. The audit showed that for the 100 records reviewed there was a 4 percent error rate. Given that the national average labor cost of each misindexed report is $200, what is the labor cost for the department for handling these misindexed reports?

    a. $8,000

    b. $500

    c. $800

    d. $500,000

59. Community Hospital discharged nine patients on April 1. The length of stay for each of the patients was as follows: patient A, 1 day; patient B, 5 days; patient C, 3 days; patient D, 3 days; patient E, 8 days; patient F, 8 days; patient G, 8 days; patient H, 9 days; patient I, 9 days. What was the average length of stay for these nine patients?

    a. Five days

    b. Six days

    c. Eight days

    d. Nine days

60. Suppose you want to display the number of deaths due to breast cancer for the years 2012 through 2022. What is the best graphic technique to use?

    a. Table

    b. Histogram

    c. Line graph

    d. Bar chart

61. Community Hospital had a total of 3,000 inpatient service days for the month of September. What was the average daily census for the hospital during September?

    a. 10 patients

    b. 96.77 patients

    c. 97 patients

    d. 100 patients

62. If an employee produces 2,080 hours of work in the course of one year, how many employees will be required for the coding area if the coding time on average for one record is 30 minutes and there are 12,500 records that must be coded each year?

    a. 3

    b. 6

    c. 36

    d. 69

63. In May, 270 women were admitted to the obstetrics service. Of these, 263 women delivered; 33 deliveries were by C-section. What is the denominator for calculating the C-section rate?

    a. 33

    b. 263

    c. 270

    d. 296

64. A health data analyst has been asked to abstract patient demographic information into an electronic database. Which of the following would the analyst include in the database?

    a. Patient date of birth

    b. Name of attending physician

    c. Patient room number

    d. Admitting diagnosis

65. A PI team is concerned with the time it is taking for patients to get through the registration process. To better understand the causes or reasons for the delay in this process the PI team would like to gather observational data. What data collection tool would be appropriate for this team to develop for their observation data?

    a. Check sheet

    b. Ordinal data tool

    c. Balance sheet

    d. Nominal data tool

66. The hospital-acquired infection rate for our hospital is 0.2%, whereas the rate at a similar hospital across town is 0.3%. This is an example of a:

    a. Benchmark

    b. Check sheet

    c. Data abstract

    d. Run chart

67. Community Hospital has been collecting quarterly data on the average monthly health record delinquency rate for the hospital. This graph depicts the trend in the delinquency rate. The hospital has established a 35 percent benchmark. Given this data, what should the hospital's Performance Improvement Council recommend?

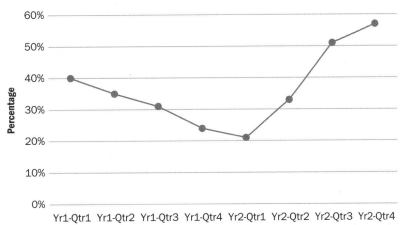

Average Monthly Medical Record Deficiency Rate

    a. Continue tracking the delinquency rate to see if the last two quarters' trend continues.

    b. Establish a higher benchmark to accommodate an increase in delinquent records.

    c. Further analyze the data to determine why the benchmark is not being met.

    d. Take an average of all the data points to arrive at a new benchmark.

68. Health departments use the health record to monitor outbreaks of diseases. In this situation what type of use of the health record does this represent?

    a. Educational

    b. Public health and research

    c. Medical review organization

    d. Patient care

69. Dr. Jones comes into the HIM department and requests that the HIM director provide a list of his records from the previous year that show a principal diagnosis of myocardial infarction. What would the HIM director use to provide this list?

    a. Disease index

    b. Master patient index

    c. Operative index

    d. Physician index

70. Community Hospital's HIM department conducted a random sample of 150 inpatient health records to determine the discharge summary completion timeliness rate. Thirteen discharges were determined to be out of compliance with completion standards. Which of the following percentages represents the timeliness rate for discharge summaries at Community Hospital?

    a. 8.7%

    b. 9.5%

    c. 41.5%

    d. 91.3%

71. Why is the MEDPAR file limited in terms of being used for research purposes?

    a. It only provides demographic data about patients.

    b. It only contains Medicare patients.

    c. It uses ICD-10-CM diagnoses and procedure codes.

    d. It breaks charges down by specific type of service.

72. In which type of distribution are the mean, median, and mode equal?

    a. Bimodal distribution

    b. Simple distribution

    c. Nonnormal distribution

    d. Normal distribution

73. In the following scatter chart what can be concluded about the relationship between age and income?

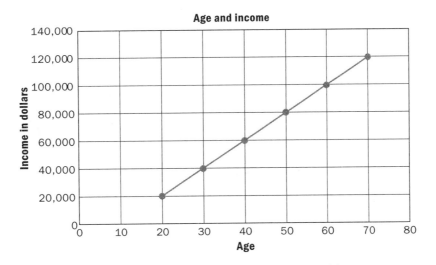

Age and income

a. There is a strong negative relationship between age and income.

b. There is no relationship between age and income.

c. There is a strong positive relationship between age and income.

d. There is not enough information to determine the relationship.

74. The facility privacy officer receives a phone call from a patient who is concerned that her former sister-in-law, a hospital employee, has accessed her health record. The privacy officer requests an audit log of activity within the patient's health record. What part of the audit log must be analyzed to determine if this complaint has merit?

a. The patient demographic information

b. Which employees viewed, created, updated, or deleted information

c. The ownership of the record

d. Whether the patient had requested to be omitted from the facility patient directory

75. General Hospital is performing peer reviews of their medical providers for quality outcomes of care. The hospital has more than 500 providers on its medical staff. The process to peer review even 10 cases for each provider is quite extensive. The quality department has concluded that to accomplish this review process, they will review 20 percent of each provider's inpatient admissions to the hospital every other year. In this situation, the quality department has applied to their review process.

a. Benchmarking

b. Data analysis

c. Sampling

d. Skewing

76. This type of chart plots all data points as a cell for two given variables of interest and, depending on frequency of observations in each cell, provides color to visualize high or low frequency.

a. Barplot

b. Scatter plot

c. Boxplot

d. Heat map

77. The process of extracting and analyzing large volumes of data from a database for the purpose of identifying hidden and sometimes subtle relationships or patterns and using those relationships to predict behaviors is called:

    a. Data mining

    b. Data warehouse

    c. Data searching

    d. Big data

78. City Hospital's Revenue Cycle Management team has established the following benchmarks: (1) The value of discharged, not final billed cases (DNFB) should not exceed two days of average daily revenue, and (2) AR days are not to exceed 60 days. The net average daily revenue is $1,000,000. The following data indicate that City Hospital's DNFB cases met its benchmarks:

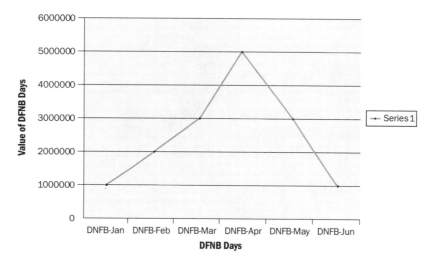

    a. 25 percent of the time

    b. 50 percent of the time

    c. 75 percent of the time

    d. 100 percent of the time

79. You are the director of HIM at Community Hospital. A physician has asked for the total number of appendectomies that he performed at your hospital last year. What type of data will you provide to the physician?

    a. Patient-specific data

    b. Aggregate data

    c. Operating room data

    d. Nothing—you cannot obtain this data after the fact

80. The director of nursing and cardiopulmonary therapy needs to know how many staff to schedule and how many ventilators will be necessary to treat the number of COVID-19 patients being admitted to ABC Hospital. You run workload and equipment projections to help determine these numbers. What type of data analytics is being performed in this scenario?

    a. Descriptive analytics

    b. Diagnostic analytics

    c. Predictive analytics

    d. Prescriptive analytics

81. The laboratory director wants the EHR to notify a physician when lab values are higher or lower than the stated normal range for this new lab test. He asks Dana to program an alert mechanism into the EHR to help physicians make quicker decisions on the patient's care. In what area of metadata is Dana functioning?

    a. Descriptive metadata

    b. Structural metadata

    c. Administrative metadata

    d. Prescriptive metadata

Domain 4 *Revenue Cycle Management*

82. A hospital can monitor its performance under the MS-DRG system by monitoring its:

    a. Accounts receivable

    b. Operating costs

    c. RBRVS payments

    d. Case-mix index

83. Which of the following is a medical condition that coexists with the primary cause of the hospitalization and affects the patient's treatment and length of stay?

    a. Case mix

    b. Complication

    c. Comorbidity

    d. Principal diagnosis

84. Patient accounting is reporting an increase in national coverage decisions (NCDs) and local coverage determinations (LCDs) failed edits in observation accounts. Which of the following departments will be tasked to resolve this issue?

    a. Health information management

    b. Patient access

    c. Patient accounts

    d. Utilization management

85. A patient is admitted to the hospital with shortness of breath and congestive heart failure. The patient subsequently develops respiratory failure. The patient undergoes intubation with ventilator management. Which of the following would be the correct sequencing and coding of this case?

    a. Congestive heart failure, respiratory failure, ventilator management, intubation

    b. Respiratory failure, intubation, ventilator management

    c. Respiratory failure, congestive heart failure, intubation, ventilator management

    d. Shortness of breath, congestive heart failure, respiratory failure, ventilator management

86. A newborn is treated for pulmonary valve stenosis, with stretching of the valve opening accomplished via a percutaneous balloon pulmonary valvuloplasty. In ICD-10-PCS, what root operation would be coded for this procedure?

    a. Alteration

    b. Dilation

    c. Repair

    d. Restriction

87. Which of the following can be used to develop a focused inpatient coding review?

    a. Controversial issues identified in *CPT Assistant*

    b. Recent data quality issues identified by external review agencies

    c. Analysis of HCPCS comparative data

    d. Top 25 APC groups by volume and charges

88. In reviewing a patient chart, the coding professional finds that the patient's chest x-ray is suggestive of chronic obstructive pulmonary disease (COPD). The attending physician mentions the x-ray finding in one progress note, but no medication, treatment, or further evaluation is provided. Which of the following actions should the coding professional take in this case?

    a. Query the attending physician and ask him to validate a diagnosis based on the chest x-ray results.

    b. Code the COPD because the documentation substantiates it.

    c. Query the radiologist to determine whether the patient has COPD.

    d. Assign a code from the abnormal findings to reflect the condition.

89. Assign codes for the following scenario: A 35-year-old male is admitted with esophageal reflux. An esophagoscopy and closed esophageal biopsy were performed.

K20.90	Esophagitis, unspecified without bleeding
K21.00	Gastro-esophageal reflux disease with esophagitis, without bleeding
K21.9	Gastro-esophageal reflux disease without esophagitis

Section	Body System	Root Operation	Body Part	Approach	Device	Qualifier
Medical and Surgical	Gastrointestinal System	Inspection	Upper Intestinal tract	Via Natural or Artificial Opening Endoscopic	No Device	No Qualifier
0	D	J	0	8	Z	Z

Section	Body System	Root Operation	Body Part	Approach	Device	Qualifier
Medical and Surgical	Gastrointestinal System	Excision	Esophagus	Via Natural or Artificial Opening Endoscopic	No Device	Diagnostic
0	D	B	5	8	Z	X

Section	Body System	Root Operation	Body Part	Approach	Device	Qualifier
Medical and Surgical	Gastrointestinal System	Excision	Esophagus	Via Natural or Artificial Opening Endoscopic	No Device	No Qualifier
0	D	B	5	8	Z	Z

a. K21.9, 0DB58ZX

b. K20.90, 0DB58ZZ

c. K21.00, 0DB58ZX

d. K21.9, 0DJ08ZZ, 0DB58ZX

90. Patient is admitted with prepatellar bursitis following a crushing injury to the left knee as a result of being hit by a car two years ago. What diagnosis codes would be assigned for this patient?

M70.40	Prepatellar bursitis, unspecified knee
M70.42	Prepatellar bursitis, left knee
S87.02XA	Crushing injury of left knee, initial encounter
S87.02XD	Crushing injury of left knee, subsequent encounter
S87.02XS	Crushing injury of left knee, sequela

a. M70.40, S87.02XA

b. M70.42, S87.02XS

c. M70.42, S87.02XD

d. M70.40, S87.02XS

91. Which of the following individuals assists in educating medical staff members on the documentation needed for accurate coding?

a. Physician champion

b. Compliance officer

c. Chargemaster coordinator

d. Data monitor

92. According to CPT, an endoscopy that is undertaken to the level of the midtransverse colon would be coded as a:

a. Proctosigmoidoscopy

b. Sigmoidoscopy

c. Colonoscopy

d. Proctoscopy

93. From the information provided, how many APCs would this patient have?

Billing Number	Status Indicator	CPT/HCPCS	APC
998323	V	99285–25	0612
998323	T	25500	0044
998323	X	72050	0261
998323	S	72128	0283
998323	S	70450	0283

a. 1

b. 4

c. 5

d. Unable to determine

94. The sum of a hospital's relative DRG weights for a year was 15,192, and the hospital had 10,471 discharges for the year. Given this information, what would be the hospital's case-mix index for that year?

    a. 0.689

    b. 0.689 × 100

    c. 1.45 × 100

    d. 1.45

95. A physician correctly prescribes Coumadin. The patient takes the Coumadin as prescribed but develops hematuria as a result of taking the medication. Which of the following is the correct way to code this case?

    a. Poisoning due to Coumadin

    b. Unspecified adverse reaction to Coumadin

    c. Hematuria; poisoning due to Coumadin

    d. Hematuria; adverse reaction to Coumadin

96. Patient had a laparoscopic incisional herniorrhaphy for a recurrent reducible hernia. The repair included insertion of mesh. What is the correct code assignment?

49560	Repair initial incisional or ventral hernia; reducible
49565	Repair recurrent incisional or ventral hernia; reducible
49568	Implantation of mesh or other prosthesis for open incisional or ventral hernia repair or mesh for closure of debridement for necrotizing soft-tissue infection
49656	Laparoscopy, surgical, repair, recurrent incisional hernia (includes mesh insertion, when performed); reducible

    a. 49565

    b. 49565, 49568

    c. 49656

    d. 49560, 49568

97. Placenta previa with delivery of twins. This patient had two prior cesarean sections. She also has a third-degree perineal laceration. This was an emergent C-section due to hemorrhage associated with the placenta previa. The appropriate principal diagnosis would be:

    a. Third-degree perineal laceration

    b. Placenta previa

    c. Twin gestation

    d. Vaginal hemorrhage

98. A patient has liver metastasis due to adenocarcinoma of the rectum. The rectum was resected two years ago. The patient has been receiving radiotherapy to the liver with some relief of pain. The patient is being admitted at this time for management of severe anemia due to the malignancy. The principal diagnosis listed on this admission is:

    a. Liver metastasis

    b. Adenocarcinoma of the rectum

    c. Anemia

    d. Admission for radiotherapy

99. Which of the following is on the list of the hospital-acquired conditions provision of the inpatient prospective payment system?

    a. Congestive heart failure

    b. Acute myocardial infarction

    c. Stage III or IV pressure ulcers

    d. Diabetic retinopathy

100. Given the information here, which of the following MS-DRGs would have the highest payment rate?

MS-DRG	MDC	Type	MS-DRG Title	Weight	Discharges	Geometric Mean	Arithmetic Mean
191	04	MED	Chronic obstructive pulmonary disease w CC	0.8843	10	2.9	3.5
192	04	MED	Chronic obstructive pulmonary disease w/o CC/MCC	0.6956	20	2.4	2.8
193	04	MED	Simple pneumonia & pleurisy w MCC	1.3120	10	4.1	5.1
194	04	MED	Simple pneumonia & pleurisy w CC	0.8639	20	3.1	3.7
195	04	MED	Simple pneumonia & pleurisy w/o CC/MCC	0.6658	10	2.5	2.9

    a. 191

    b. 192

    c. 193

    d. 194

101. Which of the following is most likely to be used in performing an outpatient coding review?

    a. OCE

    b. MS-DRG

    c. CMI

    d. MDS

102. In conducting a qualitative review, the clinical documentation specialist sees that the nursing staff has documented the patient's skin integrity on admission to support the presence of a stage I pressure ulcer. However, the physician's documentation is unclear as to whether this condition was present on admission. How should the clinical documentation specialist proceed?

    a. Note the condition as present on admission.

    b. Query the physician to determine if the condition was present on admission.

    c. Note the condition as unknown on admission.

    d. Note the condition as not present on admission.

103. The coding professional assigned separate codes for individual tests when a combination code exists. This is an example of which of the following?

    a. Upcoding

    b. Complex coding

    c. Query

    d. Unbundling

104. In a managed fee-for-service arrangement, which of the following would be used as a cost-control process for inpatient surgical services?

    a. Prospectively precertify the necessity of inpatient services

    b. Determine what services can be bundled

    c. Pay only 80 percent of the inpatient bill

    d. Require the patient to pay 20 percent of the inpatient bill

105. The patient accounting department at Wildcat Hospital is concerned because last night's bill drop contained half the usual number of inpatient cases. Which of the following reports will be most useful in determining the reason for the low volume of bills?

    a. Accounts receivable aging report

    b. Accounts not selected for billing report

    c. Case-mix index report

    d. Discharge summary report

106. The member had gastric bypass surgery three years prior. As a result of an over 200-pound weight loss, loose skin hung from the member's arms, thighs, and belly. The member, upon referral from her general surgeon, was scheduled to have a plastic surgeon to remove the excess skin. The member called for prior approval as required by the plan. The clinical review resulted in a denial of the surgery as cosmetic. The member requested a peer review and submitted documentation from her physician that the excess skin was causing skin infections and exacerbating her eczema. The peer clinician denied the case. What is the next step the member can take to have the surgery paid for by her insurance company?

    a. Appeal to the insurance company for reconsideration.

    b. Disenroll from the plan and enroll with indemnity healthcare insurance.

    c. File a lawsuit.

    d. Schedule the surgery with her original general surgeon as that surgeon was paid.

107. Which of the following coding error classifications is most valuable in determining the impact on overall revenue cycle?

    a. Errors by coding guideline

    b. Percentage of cases that could have been improved if queried

    c. Errors by coding professional

    d. Errors that produced changes in MS-DRG assignment

108. In developing an internal coding audit review program, which of the following would be risk areas that should be targeted for audit?

    a. Admission diagnosis and complaints

    b. Chargemaster description and medical necessity

    c. Clinical laboratory results

    d. Radiology orders

109. In developing a monitoring program for inpatient coding compliance, which of the following should be regularly audited?

    a. ICD-10-CM and ICD-10-PCS coding

    b. CPT/HCPCS and LOINC coding

    c. ICD-10-CM and SNOMED coding

    d. CPT/HCPCS and ICD-10-PCS coding

110. A denials management team would have which of the following goals?

    a. Identify the source of denials, improve security access controls, and develop nursing documentation.

    b. Develop nursing documentation, reduce the number of denials, and develop physician and staff knowledge of documentation, coding, and billing regulations.

    c. Identify the source of denials, reduce the number of denials, develop physician and staff knowledge of documentation, coding, and billing regulations.

    d. Reduce the number of denials, improve security access controls, and develop physician and staff knowledge of documentation, coding, and billing regulations.

111. Which of the following measures improper payments in various settings for Medicare?

    a. A/B MAC Medical Review

    b. Recovery Audit Program Contractor (RAC)

    c. Unified Program Integrity Contractor (UPIC)

    d. Comprehensive Error Rate Testing (CERT) program

112. Which of the following is an integral component of case management that helps to improve patient outcomes, lower healthcare spending, while still providing appropriate care to patients at the appropriate time?

    a. Clinical practice standards

    b. Utilization review

    c. Value-based purchasing

    d. Continuum of care review

113. Which of the following is conducted to determine if health records contain the necessary documentation, such as lab results and diagnostic test results, to support the diagnosis made by the physician?

    a. Reasonable cause

    b. Clinical validation audits

    c. Denials management

    d. Appeals management

Domain 5 *Compliance*

114. Which of the following describes incomplete records that are *not* completed by the physician within the time frame specified in the healthcare facility's policies?

    a. Suspended records

    b. Delinquent records

    c. Loose records

    d. Default records

115. The removal of medication from its usual stream of preparation, dispensing, and administration by personnel involved in those steps in order to use or sell the medication in nonhealthcare settings is called:

    a. Prescribing

    b. Adverse drug reaction

    c. Sentinel event

    d. Diversion

116. One way for a hospital to demonstrate compliance with OIG guidelines is to:

    a. Designate a privacy officer

    b. Continuously monitor PEPPER reports

    c. Develop, implement, and monitor written policies and procedures

    d. Obtain ABNs for all Medicare registrations

117. Which of the following is the principal goal of a corporate compliance program?

    a. Protect providers from sanctions or fines

    b. Increase revenues

    c. Improve patient care

    d. Limit unnecessary changes to the chargemaster

118. During an audit of health records, the HIM director finds that transcribed reports are being changed by the author up to a week after initial transcription. To remedy this situation, the HIM director should recommend which of the following?

    a. Immediately stop the practice of changing transcribed reports.

    b. Develop a facility policy that defines the acceptable period of time allowed for a transcribed document to remain in draft form.

    c. Conduct a verification audit.

    d. Alert hospital legal counsel of the practice.

119. Healthcare abuse relates to practices that may result in:

    a. False representation of fact

    b. Failure to disclose a fact

    c. Performing medically unnecessary services

    d. Knowingly submitting altered claim forms

120. A pharmacist who submits Medicaid claims for reimbursement on brand name drugs when less expensive generic drugs were dispensed has committed the crime of:

    a. Criminal negligence

    b. Fraud

    c. Perjury

    d. Products' liability

121. The HIM department has been receiving complaints about the turnaround time for release of information (ROI) requests. A PI team is created to investigate this issue. What data source would be appropriate to use to investigate this issue further?

    a. ROI employee evaluations

    b. Survey requestors

    c. ROI tracking system

    d. ADT system

122. A(n) _____ is imposed on providers by the OIG when fraud and abuse is discovered through an investigation.

    a. Corporate Integrity Agreement

    b. OIG Workplan

    c. Red Flags Rule

    d. Resource Agreement

123. The leader of the coding performance improvement team wants all her team members to clearly understand the coding process. Which of the following would be the best tool for accomplishing this objective?

    a. Scatter diagram

    b. Force-field analysis

    c. Pareto chart

    d. Flowchart

124. Recovery audit contractors (RACs) are required to have a physician medical director on staff. Additionally, RACs are charged with utilizing certified coding professionals for semi-automated and complex record reviews. Which component of the National Recovery Audit Program do these requirements support?

    a. Ensure accuracy

    b. Ensure efficiency and effectiveness

    c. Maximize transparency

    d. Minimize provider burden

125. The practice manager at the General Family Practice clinic was reviewing the established patient visit E/M code distribution for the month of May. The physicians' data is presented in the following graph. To determine the accuracy of the visit codes assigned and submitted for patients, the practice manager will need to conduct an audit of patient health records. Which physician's established patient visit code distribution should this practice manager audit as the pattern is concerning?

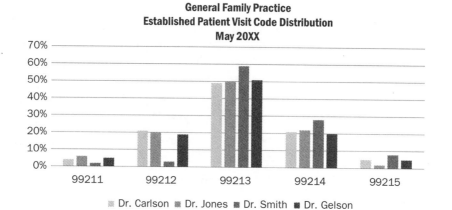

General Family Practice
Established Patient Visit Code Distribution
May 20XX

a. Dr. Carlson

b. Dr. Jones

c. Dr. Smith

d. Dr. Gelson

126. Which of the following is a fraud and abuse prevention strategy that can be used by providers to protect themselves from fraud and abuse allegations?

a. Documentation strategies

b. Strategies for noncompliance penalties

c. Strategies developed by the medical staff to enforce compliance

d. Patient readmission strategies

127. Robin is evaluating the quality of the HIE transmissions between various healthcare organizations and her healthcare organization, ABC Hospital. She is investigating the level of data and content standards' compliance to ensure that the health information transmitted to ABC Hospital is accurate, complete, comprehensive, and uncorrupted. Her job title would be:

a. Health informaticist

b. Data integrity analyst

c. Certified transfer officer

d. Systems analyst

128. Which of the following justifies the need for an external audit?

    a. It is used to appeal denials.

    b. It replaces the need for internal audits.

    c. It confirms the validity of the internal audits.

    d. It creates a one-time baseline standard.

129. Benefits of a coding compliance plan include:

    a. Retention of all coding employees

    b. Increase in denials of healthcare services reimbursement based on coding errors

    c. Elimination of errors in the health record

    d. Correction of coding-related risks

130. Which of the following is the statistical method that can be used to give every claim the same chance of being included in an audit?

    a. Systematic random sampling

    b. Simple random sampling

    c. Convenience sampling

    d. Stratified random sampling

131. Which of the following statements regarding appeal of denials is true?

    a. All types of appeals are addressed in the same way.

    b. A medical necessity appeal letter should be written by the physician.

    c. An appeal letter should be written solely by the chief compliance officer.

    d. An appeal letter should be written on all denials

132. Which of the following situations might result in a compliance audit?

    a. Low CMI

    b. High CC/MCC capture rate

    c. Decreased volume

    d. Lower reimbursement

133. A decreasing CMI is indicative of which trend?

    a. Increasing patient resource intensity

    b. Increasing proportion of surgical patients

    c. Decreasing payment per case

    d. Decreasing cost of living

Domain 6 Leadership

134. The HIM director is part of the revenue cycle management team. The discharged not final billed days are increasing because discharges are increasing. The number of coding staff is five. In an effort to increase productivity, the HIM director is researching staffing alternatives. With the implementation of an electronic document storage system, telecommuting has been suggested as an alternative. Studies report that coding productivity can increase as much as 20 percent with telecommuting. Given that discharges have increased from 100 per day to 144, how many more full-time equivalents (FTE) would need to be hired if the department went to telecommuting?

    a. 0.5 FTE

    b. 0.75 FTE

    c. 1 FTE

    d. 2 FTEs

135. Which of the following can assist managers with the tasks of monitoring productivity and forecasting budgets?

    a. Intermediary bulletins

    b. Mapping errors

    c. Revenue codes

    d. Workload statistics

136. Dr. Smith wants to use a lot of free text in his EHR. What should be your response?

    a. Good idea, Dr. Smith. This allows you to customize the documentation for each patient.

    b. Dr. Smith, we recommend that you do not use any free text in the EHR.

    c. Dr. Smith, we recommend that you should use free text only in your more complex cases.

    d. Dr. Smith, we recommend that you use little, if any, free text in the EHR.

137. An HIM department is planning to implement virtual teams for the coding and data analytics areas. Some in the facility are skeptical of this arrangement, believing that off-site employees cannot be managed. Given this work format, how can the supervisor best gauge productivity of the virtual staff?

    a. Require staff to call in to the office every morning.

    b. Require a daily conference call with all staff.

    c. Set clear goals and productivity standards and see that these are met.

    d. Install camcorders on each team member's computer to ensure that they are at their workstations.

138. Which of the following strategies would be best to ensure that all stakeholders are engaged in the planning and development of an organization EHR system?

    a. Form an EHR steering committee.

    b. Put out a press release.

    c. Distribute an organization-wide memorandum from the CEO.

    d. Put out a notice on the organization's intranet.

139. An HIM department has set productivity standards for each task associated with scanning records of discharged patients. The standard for the scanning process is 1,500 images per hour worked. Twelve weeks after implementation, the standard is reassessed because of errors made by some employees. Given this data, what action might the HIM manager or director want to take regarding quality of production?

Employee Scanning Productivity			
Employee	**Actual Production**	**Hours Worked**	**Percentage Errors**
Chad	1,325 images/hour	242	1%
Barbara	1,500 images/hour	240	2%
Leslie	1,450 images/hour	232	1%
Maria	1,700 image/hour	240	7%
Mike	1,675 images/hour	220	6%

   a. Talk with Chad and put him on probation for not meeting the productivity standard.

   b. Complement Maria and Mike for exceeding the productivity standard.

   c. Incorporate quality expectations into the standard.

   d. Continue to benchmark another six weeks to see if there is any difference.

140. The manager calculated a unit and time productivity statistic based on employee self-reported data. Which method did he use to develop this performance standard?

   a. Benchmarking

   b. Work distribution analysis

   c. Work measurement

   d. Workflow analysis

141. An HIM supervisor is revising job descriptions for record scanning positions. These positions have been in existence for just over one year. Which of the following would be the most appropriate action to take to ensure all tasks being performed are included in the new job descriptions?

   a. Ask current staff members to keep a diary for a certain period of time on how they spend their time.

   b. Review job descriptions from other hospitals.

   c. Make random observations of job tasks.

   d. Refer the matter to the human resources department.

142. Dr. Wilson asks you, the EHR manager, to explain the difference between an alert and a reminder. You explain that reminders are typically used for things that can be scheduled or that occur on a regular basis. An example of a reminder that would be given to Dr. Wilson would be:

   a. Use of anticoagulant is contraindicated.

   b. Patient is due for MMR immunization.

   c. Patient is allergic to sulfa drugs.

   d. Drug does not come in this format.

143. A hospital currently uses the patient's Social Security number as their patient identifier. The hospital risk manager has identified this as a potential identity fraud risk and wants the information removed. The risk manager is not getting cooperation from the physicians and others in the hospital who say they need the information for identification and other purposes. Given this situation, what should the HIM director suggest?

    a. Avoid displaying the number on any document, screen, or data collection field.

    b. Allow the information in both electronic and paper forms since a variety of people need this data.

    c. Require employees to sign confidentiality agreements if they have access to Social Security numbers.

    d. Contact legal counsel for advice.

144. Which phase in the project life cycle is where the project shifts to become an integrated part of organizational operations?

    a. Closure

    b. Execution

    c. Initiation

    d. Planning

145. City Hospital's HIPAA committee is considering a change in policy to allow hospital employees who are also hospital patients to access their own patient information in the hospital's EHR system. A committee member notes that HIPAA provides rights to patients to view their own health information. However, another member wonders if this action might present other problems. In this situation, what information should the HIM director provide?

    a. HIPAA requires that employees have access to their own information, so grant privileges to the employees to perform this function.

    b. HIPAA does not allow employees to have access to their own information, so the procedure should not be implemented.

    c. Allowing employees to access their own records using their job-based access rights appears to violate HIPAA's minimum necessary requirement; therefore, allow employees to access their records through normal procedures.

    d. Employees are considered a special class of people under HIPAA and the procedure should be implemented.

146. City Hospital has implemented a procedure that allows inpatients to decide whether they want to be listed in the hospital's directory. The directory information includes the patient's name, location in the hospital, and general condition. If a patient elects to be in the directory, this information is used to inform callers who know the patient's name. Some patients have requested that they be listed in the directory, but information is to be released to only a list of specific people the patient provides. A hospital committee is considering changing the policy to accommodate these types of patients. In this case, what type of advice should the HIM director provide?

    a. Approve the requests because this is a patient right under HIPAA regulations.

    b. Deny these requests because screening of calls is difficult to manage and if information is given in error, this would be considered a violation of HIPAA.

    c. Develop two different types of directories—one directory for provision of all information and one directory for provision of information to selected friends and family of the patient.

    d. Deny these requests and seek approval from the Office for Civil Rights.

147. The cardiologist group wants to add some terms and abbreviations that have been developed in their clinic. Their IT coordinator comes to you and asks to put these into the EHR system. You inform him that these must be recognized and meet standard requirements of the most widely recognized nomenclature in healthcare, which is:

    a. ICD-10

    b. ICD-9

    c. SNOMED-CT

    d. ANSI

148. To develop performance standards for release of information turnaround time, the manager conducted a literature search and contacted peer institutions. Which method did she use?

    a. Benchmarking

    b. Workflow analysis

    c. Productivity analysis

    d. Work measurement

149. At which stage in project management process would the status of the project be assessed regularly in reference to planned activities and their timeline, and if the project is off target, a project manager would take action to bring it back on track?

    a. Controlling and monitoring

    b. Execution

    c. Initiation

    d. Planning

150. If steps in a revenue cycle process are handled separately in sequence by individual workers, the method of organizing work is called which of the following?

    a. Serial work division

    b. Parallel work division

    c. Processing

    d. Benchmarking

PRACTICE QUESTIONS

Domain 1 *Data Content, Structure, and Information Governance*

1. In healthcare, data sets serve two purposes. The first is to identify data elements to be collected about each patient. The second is to:

    a. Provide uniform data definitions

    b. Guide connection between two systems

    c. Guide access to data that exists in multiple databases

    d. Provide a research database

2. A health information technician is responsible for designing a data collection form to collect data on patients in an acute-care hospital. The first resource that she should use is:

    a. ORYX

    b. UACDS

    c. MDS

    d. UHDDS

3. To help support and manage data elements within an electronic health record (EHR) the organization should implement a to support standardized input and understanding of all data elements.

    a. Data map

    b. Core content

    c. Clinical repository

    d. Data dictionary

4. Reviewing a health record for missing signatures and medical reports is called:

    a. Analysis

    b. Coding

    c. Assembly

    d. Indexing

5. Which of the following is *not* a characteristic of the common healthcare data sets such as UHDDS and UACDS?

    a. They define minimum data elements to be collected.

    b. They provide a complete and exhaustive list of data elements that must be collected.

    c. They provide a framework for data collection to which an individual facility can add data items.

    d. They vary by their purpose and use.

6. Ensuring data are not altered during transmission across a network or during storage is called:

    a. Media control

    b. Audit controls

    c. Mitigation

    d. Integrity

7. The primary purpose of a data set in healthcare is to:

    a. Recommend common data elements to be collected in health records

    b. Mandate all data that must be contained in a health record

    c. Define reportable data for federally funded programs

    d. Standardize medical vocabulary

8. A notation for a diabetic patient in a physician progress note reads: "Occasionally gets hungry. No insulin reactions. She says she is following her diabetic diet." In which part of a problem-oriented health record progress note would this be written?

    a. Subjective

    b. Objective

    c. Assessment

    d. Plan

9. An audit of a hospital's electronic health system shows that diagnostic codes are not being reported at the correct level of detail. This indicates a problem with data:

    a. Consistency

    b. Granularity

    c. Comprehensiveness

    d. Relevancy

10. In which of the following examples does the gender of the patient constitute information rather than a data element?

    a. As an entry to be completed on the face sheet of the health record

    b. In the note "50-year-old white male" in the patient history

    c. In a study comparing the incidence of myocardial infarctions in black males as compared to white females

    d. In a study of the age distribution of lung cancer patients

11. Which of the following is a core data set developed by ASTM to communicate a patient's past and current health information as the patient transitions from one care setting to another?

    a. Ambulatory Care Data Set

    b. Continuity of Care Document

    c. Minimum Data Set

    d. Uniform Hospital Discharge Data Set

12. Which of the following data sets does the home health prospective payment system use for patient assessments?

    a. HEDIS

    b. OASIS

    c. MDS

    d. UHDDS

13. A notation for a hypertensive patient in a physician ambulatory care progress note reads: "Blood pressure adequately controlled." In which part of a problem-oriented health record progress note would this be written?

    a. Assessment

    b. Objective

    c. Plan

    d. Subjective

14. During a review of documentation practices, the HIM director finds that nurses are routinely using the copy and paste functionality of the hospital's EHR system for documenting nursing notes. Which of the following should the HIM director do to ensure that the nurses are following acceptable documentation practices?

    a. Inform the nurses that copy and paste is not acceptable and to stop this practice immediately.

    b. Determine how many nurses are involved in this practice.

    c. Institute an in-service training session on documentation practices.

    d. Develop policy and procedures related to cutting, copying, and pasting documentation in the EHR system.

15. The data set designed to organize data about public health issues to inform purchasers and consumers about the performance of healthcare plans is:

    a. UHDDS

    b. DEEDS

    c. MDS

    d. HEDIS

16. Joe Clark's admitting data indicates that her birth date is March 21, 1948. On the discharge summary, Joe's birth date is recorded as July 21, 1948. Which quality element is missing from Joe's health record?

    a. Data completeness

    b. Data consistency

    c. Data accessibility

    d. Data comprehensiveness

17. Identify where the following information would be found in the acute-care record: "Following induction of an adequate general anesthesia, and with the patient supine on the padded table, the left upper extremity was prepped and draped in the standard fashion."

    a. Anesthesia report

    b. Physician progress notes

    c. Operative report

    d. Recovery room record

18. Which of the following are clear guidelines for the acceptable values of specific data fields and making exchange health information using electronic networks possible?

    a. Data content standards

    b. Messaging standards

    c. Interoperability standards

    d. Vocabulary standards

19. In long-term care, the resident's care plan is based on data collected in the:

    a. UHDDS

    b. OASIS

    c. MDS

    d. HEDIS

20. Which of the following is a primary purpose of the health record?

    a. Document patient care delivery

    b. Regulation of healthcare facilities

    c. Aid in education of nurses and physicians

    d. Assist in process redesign

21. Which of the following best describes data accessibility?

    a. Data are correct.

    b. Data are easy to obtain.

    c. Data include all required elements.

    d. Data are reliable.

22. A physician is reviewing the lab results of a patient in his office. The EHR screen displays one set of results in red with a flashing asterisk and also shows that this result is three times higher than the expected value. This is an example of a(n):

    a. Alert

    b. Audit

    c. Structured data

    d. Unstructured data

23. Identify where the following documentation would be found in the acute-care record: "CBC: WBC 12.0, RBC 4.65, HGB 14.8, HCT 43.3, MCV 93."

    a. Laboratory report

    b. Pathology report

    c. Physical examination

    d. Physician orders

24. The attending physician is responsible for which of the following types of acute-care documentation?

    a. Consultation report

    b. Discharge summary

    c. Laboratory report

    d. Pathology report

25. Which of the following represents an example of data granularity?

    a. A progress note recorded at or near the time of the observation

    b. An acceptable range of values defined for a clinical characteristic

    c. A numerical measurement carried out to the appropriate decimal place

    d. A health record that includes all of the required components

26. Which of the following is an example of clinical data?

    a. Admitting diagnosis

    b. Date and time of admission

    c. Insurance information

    d. Health record number

27. Dr. Jones entered a progress note in a patient's health record 24 hours after he visited the patient. Which quality element is missing from the progress note?

    a. Data completeness

    b. Data relevancy

    c. Data currency

    d. Data precision

28. In which department or unit is the health record number typically assigned?

    a. HIM

    b. Patient registration

    c. Nursing

    d. Billing

29. The following is documented in an acute-care record: "Spoke to the attending re: my assessment. Provided adoption and counseling information. Spoke to CPS re: referral. Case manager to meet with patient and family." In which of the following would this documentation appear?

    a. Admission note

    b. Dietary note

    c. Physician progress note

    d. Social service note

30. Deficiencies in a health record include which of the following?

    a. Contradictory content

    b. Mistake in the patient's age

    c. Illegible content

    d. Missing document

31. In preparation for her annual physical, Amanda uploads her diet and fitness log from her smartwatch, and adds information about her previous medical history for her physician to review. Amanda is using what type of software application offered by her provider's practice?

    a. Patient portal

    b. Scheduling system

    c. Computerized provider order entry

    d. E-prescribing system

32. Which of the following represents documentation of the patient's current and past health status?

    a. Physical exam

    b. Medical history

    c. Physician orders

    d. Patient consent

33. A nurse is responsible for which of the following types of acute-care documentation?

    a. Medication administration record

    b. Radiology report

    c. Operative report

    d. Therapy assessment

34. What is the function of a consultation report?

    a. Provides a chronological summary of the patient's medical history and illness

    b. Documents opinions about the patient's condition from the perspective of a physician not previously involved in the patient's care

    c. Concisely summarizes the patient's treatment and stay in the hospital

    d. Documents the physician's instructions to other parties involved in providing care to a patient

35. A secondary purpose of the health record is to provide support for which of the following?

    a. Provider reimbursement

    b. Education for patients

    c. Research activities

    d. Delivery of patient care

36. The following is documented in an acute-care record: "HEENT: Reveals the tympanic membranes, nares, and pharynx to be clear. No obvious head trauma. CHEST: Good bilateral chest sounds." In which of the following would this documentation appear?

    a. Medical history

    b. Pathology report

    c. Operation report

    d. Physical examination

37. What term describes the processing of scanning past health records into the information system so there is an existing database of patient information, making the information system valuable to the user?

    a. Abstracting

    b. Analysis

    c. Backscanning

    d. Barcoding

38. What makes the indexing of scanned health record more efficient because it can enter metadata automatically?

    a. Barcodes

    b. Interoperability

    c. Scanning

    d. Deficiency management

39. Two HIM professionals are abstracting data for the same case for a registry. When their work is checked, discrepancies are found. Which data quality component is lacking?

    a. Completeness

    b. Validity

    c. Reliability

    d. Timeliness

40. "I have recommended to Mr. Palmer that we proceed with CT scan of head to rule out bleed. Thank you for allowing me to participate in Mr. Palmer's care today." This documentation would be found in which type of report?

    a. Consultation report

    b. Operative report

    c. Pathology report

    d. Anesthesia report

41. Which of the following contains the physician's findings based on an examination of the patient?

    a. Physical exam

    b. Discharge summary

    c. Medical history

    d. Patient instructions

42. Which of the following best describes data comprehensiveness?

    a. Data are correct.

    b. Data are easy to obtain.

    c. Data include all required elements.

    d. Data are reliable.

43. Which database must a healthcare facility query as part of the credentialing process when a physician initially applies for medical staff privileges?

    a. UHDDS

    b. NPDB

    c. MEDPAR

    d. HEDIS

44. How are amendments handled in the EHR?

    a. Amendments are automatically appended to the original note. No additional signature is required.

    b. Amendments must be entered by the same person as the original note.

    c. Amendments cannot be entered after 24 hours of the event.

    d. The amendment must have separate authentication, date, and time.

45. Which of the following is an example of individual user of the health record?

    a. Accreditation organization

    b. Policy-making body

    c. Government licensing agency

    d. Patient

46. HIM departments may be the hub of identifying, mitigating, and correcting MPI errors, but that information often is not shared with other departments within the healthcare organization. After identifying procedural problems with admitting patients that contribute to the creation of the MPI errors, which department should the MPI manager work with to correct these procedural problems?

    a. Administration

    b. Registration

    c. Risk Management

    d. Radiology and Laboratory

47. The HIM analyst is noticing that the progress notes documented by Dr. Stevens are repetitive and very similar. Which of the following terms identifies the type of documentation issue being used by Dr. Stevens?

    a. Case-mix index

    b. Key indicator

    c. Copy and paste functionality

    d. Retrospective query

48. The coding manager at Community Hospital is seeing an increased number of physicians failing to document the cause and effect of diabetes and its manifestations. Which of the following will provide the most comprehensive solution to handle this documentation issue?

    a. Instruct coding professionals to continue querying the attending physician for this documentation.

    b. Present this information at the next medical staff meeting to inform physicians on documentation standards and guidelines.

    c. Do nothing because coding compliance guidelines do not allow any action.

    d. Place all offending physicians on suspension if the documentation issues continue.

49. Which of the following elements of coding quality represent the degree to which codes accurately reflect the patient's diagnoses and procedures?

    a. Reliability

    b. Validity

    c. Completeness

    d. Timeliness

50. OASIS data are used to assess the _____ of home health services.

    a. Core measure

    b. Financial performance

    c. Outcome

    d. Utilization

51. The act of granting approval to a healthcare organization based on whether the organization has met a set of voluntary standards is called:

    a. Accreditation

    b. Licensure

    c. Acceptance

    d. Approval

52. Which of the following has been responsible for accrediting healthcare organizations since the mid-1950s and determines whether the organization is continually monitoring and improving the quality of care provided?

    a. Commission on Accreditation of Rehabilitation Facilities

    b. American Osteopathic Association

    c. National Committee for Quality Assurance

    d. Joint Commission

53. What committee usually oversees the development and approval of new forms for the health record?

    a. Clinical forms committee

    b. Executive committee

    c. Medical staff committee

    d. Quality review committee

54. The medical staff at University Medical Center is nationally renowned for its skill in performing cardiac procedures. The nursing staff in the cardiac unit has noticed that a significant number of health records do not have informed consents prior to the performance of procedures. Obtaining informed consent is the responsibility of the:

    a. Administration

    b. Nursing staff

    c. Admissions department

    d. Physician

55. Which specialized type of progress note provides healthcare professionals impressions of patient problems with detailed treatment action steps?

    a. Flow record

    b. Vital signs record

    c. Care plan

    d. Surgical note

56. When meeting with the HIM professional during an on-site review, the surveyor would be looking for what type of information?

    a. Written policies and procedures on document imaging

    b. HIM department's success in documentation compliance

    c. Document type matrix

    d. Attendance policy

57. What is the private, not-for-profit organization committed to developing and maintaining practical, customer-focused standards to help organizations measure and improve the quality, value, and outcomes of behavioral health and medical rehabilitation programs?

    a. Commission on Accreditation of Rehabilitation Facilities

    b. American Osteopathic Association

    c. National Committee for Quality Assurance

    d. Joint Commission

58. Multiple users entering data may have different definitions or perceptions about what goes into a data field, thereby confounding the data. For example, one department may use the term *patient* while another department my use the term *client* to define the same entity. Which of the following would be used to provide standardization?

    a. Data dictionary

    b. Data mining

    c. Data model

    d. Database

59. Which accrediting organization has instituted continuous improvement and sentinel event monitoring, and uses tracer methodology during survey visits?

    a. Accreditation Association for Ambulatory Healthcare

    b. Commission on Accreditation of Rehabilitation Facilities

    c. American Osteopathic Association

    d. Joint Commission

60. The ability to electronically send data from one information system to another while maintaining the original meaning is called:

    a. Data comparability

    b. Interoperability

    c. National data exchange

    d. Data architecture

61. What is the key piece of data needed to link a patient's information who is seen in a variety of care settings?

    a. Facility medical record number

    b. Facility identification number

    c. Identity matching algorithm

    d. Patient birth date

62. Which of the following is *not* true of good electronic forms design?

    a. Minimizes keystrokes by using pop-up menus

    b. Performs completeness check for all required data

    c. Uses radio buttons to select multiple items from a set of options

    d. Uses text boxes to enter text

63. Which of the following is necessary to ensure that each term used in an EHR has a common meaning to all users?

    a. Controlled vocabulary

    b. Data exchange standards

    c. Encoded vocabulary

    d. Proprietary standards

64. What is the primary benefit of point-of-care documentation?

    a. Eases duplicate data entry burden

    b. Eliminates intermediary paper forms

    c. Eliminates the need for provider documentation

    d. Ensures that appropriate data are collected timely

65. When a user keys in 10101963, the computer displays it as 10/10/1963. What enables this?

    a. Toolkit

    b. Input mask

    c. Check box

    d. Radio button

66. What is the term used to identify a separate database or system within a department that does not integrate into the main organizational system nor can it be accessed by others outside that specific department?

    a. Information silo

    b. Information system

    c. Information technology

    d. Information architecture

67. Specific performance expectations, structures, and processes that provide detailed information and the intent for each of the Joint Commission standards are called:

    a. Elements of performance

    b. Fact sheets

    c. Ad hoc reports

    d. Registers

68. When all required data elements are included in the health record, the quality characteristic for data _____ is met.

    a. Security

    b. Accessibility

    c. Flexibility

    d. Comprehensiveness

69. A record that fails quantitative analysis is missing the quality criterion of:

    a. Legibility

    b. Reliability

    c. Completeness

    d. Clarity

70. Which data set was developed by the National Committee for Quality Assurance to aid consumers with health-related issues with information to compare performance of clinical measures for health plans?

    a. HEDIS

    b. UHDDS

    c. UACDS

    d. ORYX

71. Joan reviewed the health record of Sally Williams and found the physician stated on her post-op note, "examined after surgery." This review process would be an example of:

    a. Quantitative analysis

    b. Qualitative analysis

    c. Data mining

    d. Data warehousing

72. Which of the following data sets would be most useful in developing a matrix for identification of components of the legal health record?

    a. Document name, media type, source system, electronic storage start date, stop printing start date

    b. Document name, media type

    c. Document name, medical record number, source system

    d. Document name, source system

73. Authentication of a record refers to:

    a. Establishment of its baseline trustworthiness

    b. The type of electronic operating system on which it was created

    c. The identity of the individual who notarized it

    d. Its relevance

74. The following descriptors about the data element PATIENT_LAST_NAME are included in a data dictionary—definition: legal surname of the patient; field type: numeric; field length: 50; required field: yes; default value: none; input mask: none. Which of the following is true about the definition of this data element?

    a. The field type should be changed to alphanumeric.

    b. The input mask should be changed from None to Required.

    c. The field length should be shortened.

    d. A default value should be Required.

75. General documentation guidelines apply to:

    a. Only electronic health records

    b. All categories of health records

    c. All emergency health records

    d. Only paper-based health records

76. What type of health records may contain family and caregiver input?

    a. Behavioral health records

    b. Ambulatory surgery health records

    c. Emergency department health records

    d. Obstetric health record

77. Why should the copy and paste function not be used in the electronic health record?

    a. The content may contain outdated information.

    b. Joint Commission standards prevent this practice.

    c. This feature is never found in the electronic health record.

    d. Medicare has a regulation against this practice.

78. An RAI/MDS and care plan are found in records of patients in what setting?

    a. Home healthcare

    b. Long-term care

    c. Behavioral healthcare

    d. Rehabilitative care

79. The evaluation of data collected based on business needs and strategy is part of:

    a. Data ownership

    b. Data stewardship

    c. Data quality

    b. Data modeling

80. A patient's birth date and gender documented in the health record are examples of a data:

    a. Element

    b. Map

    c. Dictionary

    d. Definition

81. Which Joint Commission survey methodology involves an evaluation that follows the hospital experiences of past or current patients?

    a. Priority focus process review

    b. Periodic performance review

    c. Tracer methodology

    d. Performance improvement

82. George reviewed the patient record of Mr. Brown and found there was no H&P on the record at seven hours past this patient's admission time. This review process would be an example of:

    a. Data mining

    b. Qualitative analysis

    c. Quantitative analysis

    d. Data warehousing

83. In a cancer registry, the accession number:

    a. Identifies all the cases of cancer treated in a given year

    b. Is the number assigned to each case as it is entered into a cancer registry

    c. Identifies the pathologic diagnosis of an individual cancer

    d. Is the number assigned for the diagnosis of a cancer patient that is entered into the cancer registry treatments and at different stages of cancer

84. Bob Smith is a 56-year-old white male. This is an example of what type of data?

    a. Secondary

    b. Primary

    c. Aggregate

    d. Patient-identifiable

85. What type of registry maintains a database of patients injured by an external physical force?

    a. Implant registry

    b. Birth defects registry

    c. Trauma registry

    d. Transplant registry

86. Which of the following describe criteria with specific objectives and measures that hospitals must meet to demonstrate they are using EHRs that positively affect patient care?

    a. Approved certified EHR technology

    b. Hospital standardization program

    c. Quality improvement standards

    d. Promoting interoperability program

87. Which of the following systems is the key to identifying a patient's multiple hospitalizations?

    a. CDR

    b. CPOE

    c. MPI

    d. R-ADT

88. Which of the following would be used to track data movement from one system to another?

    a. Administrative metadata

    b. Business metadata

    c. Context metadata

    d. Embedded metadata

89. The statement, "the unique patient identifier must be numeric," is an example of which of the following business rule categories?

    a. Constraint

    b. Definition

    c. Derivation

    d. Relational

90. Which of the following is the best definition of a forward map in data mapping?

    a. Linking of two systems in the opposite direction

    b. Linking an older version of a code set to a newer version

    c. Linking a newer version of a code set to an older version

    d. Linking a source system to a target system

91. The patient's address is the same in the master patient index, electronic health record, laboratory information system, and other systems. This means that the data values are consistent and therefore indicative of which of the following?

    a. Data availability

    b. Data accessibility

    c. Data privacy

    d. Data integrity

92. The term used to describe controlling information is:

    a. Information power

    b. Information authority

    c. Information governance

    d. Information policy

93. Which of the following data quality characteristics means all data items are included within the information collected?

    a. Accuracy

    b. Consistency

    c. Comprehensiveness

    d. Relevancy

94. When creating guidelines of health record documentation, which of the following should be evaluated?

    a. The personal preferences of the healthcare practitioner

    b. The documentation needs based on accreditation standards

    c. Information taught in the local nursing programs

    d. The wants of the department chairs in a hospital

95. The use of the health record by a clinician to facilitate quality patient care is considered:

    a. A primary purpose of the health record

    b. Patient care support

    c. A secondary purpose of the health record

    d. Patient care effectiveness

96. Which group focuses on accreditation of rehabilitation programs and services?

    a. HFAP

    b. Joint Commission

    c. AAAHC

    d. CARF

97. What is it called when accrediting bodies, such as the Joint Commission, rather than the government can survey facilities for compliance with the Medicare Conditions of Participation for Hospitals?

    a. Deemed status

    b. Licensure

    c. Subpoena

    d. Credentialing

98. Which of the following statements represents knowledge?

    a. Hematocrit is 48 today.

    b. Mary Jones had a blood pressure of 120/100.

    c. The hospital has an 89 percent occupancy rate.

    d. Mary Jones's hemoglobin of 13 is within normal range.

99. Results of a urinalysis and all blood tests performed would be found in what part of a healthcare record?

    a. Autopsy report

    b. Laboratory report

    c. Pathology report

    d. Surgical report

100. Which of the following is considered a clinical documentation best practice?

    a. Allowing clinicians to backdate physician orders

    b. Restricting use of abbreviations to a list approved by hospital and medical staff bylaws, rules, and regulations

    c. Allowing clinicians to delete documentation errors in an electronic record

    d. Prohibiting all verbal orders

101. Dr. Hall is an orthopedic surgeon performing a knee replacement on Mary. Mary was seen in Dr. Hall's office two months before the surgery and Dr. Hall documented her history and physical (H&P) at that point. Does this H&P meet documentation requirements for the surgery?

    a. No, the first H&P must be documented within 60 days before admission, and another H&P must be documented within 48 hours after admission to the hospital.

    b. Yes, there are no requirements on when an H&P must be performed.

    c. No, the H&P must be documented within 30 days before admission with an update within 24 hours after admission.

    d. Yes, because the H&P was documented within 60 days.

102. A patient's registration forms, personal property list, RAI, care plan, and discharge or transfer documentation would be found most frequently in which type of health record?

    a. Rehabilitative care

    b. Ambulatory care

    c. Behavioral health

    d. Long-term care

103. Max Fields receives an email alert to check his MyRecord account. When Max checks this account, he has a notification from his doctor to schedule his annual physical. This type of encounter is via the use of a:

    a. Health information exchange

    b. Clinical decision support system

    c. Patient portal

    d. Electronic information system

104. Electronic systems used by nurses and physicians to document assessments and findings are called:

    a. Computerized provider order entry

    b. Electronic document management systems

    c. Medication administration record

    d. Point-of-care charting

105. Which of the following is *not* part of data governance?

    a. Ensuring control and accountability for enterprise data

    b. Establishing and monitoring data policies

    c. Assigning data decision rights and accountabilities for data

    d. Promoting the sale of enterprise data

106. A healthcare system wants to map ICD-10-CM to ICD-9-CM. Which of the following would be true about this effort?

    a. ICD-10-CM would be considered the target system.

    b. This is an example of reverse mapping.

    c. This is an example of forward mapping.

    d. This is an example of bidirectional mapping.

107. What is the primary purpose of structured data entry?

    a. Provide providers with as many options as possible

    b. Speed up data entry

    c. Reduce documentation variability

    d. Comply with regulatory rules

108. A deterministic algorithm would use which of the following data elements to disqualify two or more similar records?

    a. Phone number

    b. Date of birth

    c. Email address

    d. Last name

109. In data matching which of the following best describes an overlap?

    a. When one entity in a database has multiple unique identifiers

    b. When one entity is assigned another entity's unique identifier

    c. When one entity has different unique identifiers in different databases

    d. When one database overlaps with another database

110. Which of the following should be taken into consideration when designing a health record form?

    a. Including original and revised dates

    b. Number of clicks to access data

    c. Choosing the field type such as radio buttons

    d. Difference between paper and screen

Domain 2 *Access, Disclosure, Privacy, and Security*

111. Which of the following is an example of data security?

    a. Contingency planning

    b. Fire protection

    c. Automatic log-off after inactivity

    d. Key card for access to data center

112. Which of the following is *not* an automatic control that helps preserve data confidentiality and integrity in an electronic system?

    a. Edit checks

    b. Audit trails

    c. Password management

    d. Security awareness program

113. "Our computer system notified us that Mary Burchfield just looked up another patient with the same last name." This notification is called a(n):

    a. Trigger

    b. Audit reduction tool

    c. Integrity

    d. Audit control

114. How long should the MPI be retained?

    a. Permanently

    b. 10 years

    c. 25 years

    d. 50 years

115. An audit trail may be used to detect which of the following?

    a. Unauthorized access to a system

    b. Loss of data

    c. Presence of a virus

    d. Successful completion of a backup

116. Which of the following administrative safeguards includes policies and procedures for responding to emergencies or failures in systems that contain e-PHI?

    a. A contingency plan

    b. Security training

    c. Workforce security

    d. Information access management

117. Which of the following statements is true in regard to responding to requests from individuals for access to their protected health information (PHI)?

    a. A cost-based fee may be charged for retrieval of the PHI.

    b. A cost-based fee may be charged for making a copy of the PHI.

    c. No fees of any type may be charged.

    d. A minimal fee may be charged for retrieval and copying of PHI.

118. Under HIPAA rules, when an individual asks to see his or her own health information, a covered entity:

    a. Must always provide access

    b. Can always deny access

    c. Can demand that the individual pay to see his or her record

    d. Can deny access to psychotherapy notes

119. In which of the following situations must a covered entity provide an appeals process for denials to requests from individuals to see their own health information?

    a. Any time access is requested

    b. When the covered entity is a correctional institution

    c. When a licensed healthcare professional has determined that access to PHI would likely endanger the life or safety of the individual

    d. When the covered entity is unable to produce the health record

120. Within the context of electronic health records, protecting data privacy means defending or safeguarding:

    a. Access to information

    b. Data availability

    c. Health record quality

    d. System implementation

121. To ensure relevancy, an organization's security policies and procedures should be reviewed at least:

    a. Once every six months

    b. Once a year

    c. Every two years

    d. Every five years

122. An electronic health record risk analysis is useful to:

    a. Identify security threats

    b. Identify which employees should have access to data

    c. Establish password controls

    d. Establish audit controls

123. An individual designated as an inpatient coding professional may have access to an electronic health record to code the record. Under what access security mechanism is the coding professional allowed access to the system?

    a. Situation-based

    b. User-based

    c. Context-based

    d. Role-based

124. Which of the following are policies and procedures required by HIPAA that address the management of computer resources and security?

    a. Access controls

    b. Administrative safeguards

    c. Audit safeguards

    d. Role-based controls

125. What is the biggest threat to the security of healthcare data?

    a. Natural disasters

    b. Fires

    c. Employees

    d. Equipment malfunctions

126. The protection measures and tools for safeguarding information and information systems is a definition of:

    a. Confidentiality

    b. Data security

    c. Informational privacy

    d. Informational access control

127. The HIM supervisor suspects that a departmental employee is accessing the EHR for personal reasons, but has no specific data to support this suspicion. In this case, what should the supervisor do?

    a. Confront the employee.

    b. Send out a memorandum to all department employees reminding them of the hospital policy on internet use.

    c. Ask the security officer for audit trail data to confirm or disprove the suspicion.

    d. Transfer the employee to another job that does not require computer usage.

128. Placing locks on computer room doors is considered what type of security control?

    a. Access control

    b. Workstation control

    c. Physical safeguard

    d. Security breach

129. The administrative assistant in the hospital Radiology Department was recently hospitalized with ketoacidosis. She comes to the HIM department and requests to review her health record. Which of the following is the best course of action?

    a. Allow her to review her record after obtaining authorization from her.

    b. Refer the patient to her physician for the information.

    c. Tell her to go through her supervisor for the information.

    d. Tell her that hospital employees cannot access their own medical records.

130. St. Joseph's Hospital has a psychiatric service on the sixth floor of the hospital. A 31-year-old male has come to the HIM department and requested to see a copy of his medical record. He indicated he was a patient of Dr. Schmidt, a psychiatrist, and that he was on the sixth floor of St. Joseph's for the past two months. These records are not psychotherapy notes. Which of the following is the best course of action?

    a. Prohibit the patient from accessing his record, as it contains psychiatric diagnoses that may greatly upset him.

    b. Allow the patient to access his record.

    c. Allow the patient to access his record if, after contacting his physician, his physician does not think it will be harmful to the patient.

    d. Deny access because HIPAA prevents patients from reviewing their psychiatric records.

131. During user acceptance testing of a new EHR system, physicians are complaining that they must use multiple log-on screens to access all the system modules. For example, they must use one log-on for CPOE and another log-on to view laboratory results. One physician suggests having a single sign-on that would provide access to all the EHR system components. However, the hospital administrator thinks that one log-on would be a security issue. What information should the HIM director provide?

    a. Single sign-on is not supported by HIPAA security measures.

    b. Single sign-on is discouraged by the Joint Commission.

    c. Single sign-on is less frustrating for the end user and can provide better security.

    d. Single sign-on is not possible given today's technology.

132. Which of the following are security safeguards that protect equipment, media, and facilities?

    a. Administrative controls

    b. Physical safeguards

    c. Audit controls

    d. Role based safeguards

133. What does the term *access control* mean?

    a. Identifying the greatest security risks

    b. Identifying which data employees should have a right to use

    c. Implementing safeguards that protect physical media

    d. Restricting access to computer rooms and facilities

134. What resource should be consulted in terms of who may authorize access, use, or disclose the health records of minors?

    a. HIPAA, because it has strict rules regarding minors.

    b. Hospital attorneys, because they know the rules of the hospital.

    c. State law, because HIPAA defers to state laws on matters related to minors.

    d. Federal law, because HIPAA overrides state laws on matters related to minors.

135. A secure method of communication between the healthcare provider and the patient is a(n):

    a. Personal health record

    b. Email

    c. Patient portal

    d. Online health information

136. The director of health information services is allowed access to the health record tracking system when providing the proper log-in and password. What is this access security mechanism called?

    a. Context-based

    b. User-based

    c. Situation-based

    d. Application-based

137. A special web page that offers secure access to data is a(n):

    a. Internet

    b. Home page

    c. Intranet

    d. Portal

138. A provider's office inadvertently shared Mary's PHI with another patient. Which of the following breach notification statements is correct regarding the physician office's required action?

    a. It must report the breach to HHS within 60 days after the end of the calendar year in which the breach occurred.

    b. It must report the breach to HHS within 60 days of the breach.

    c. It must notify all local media outlets and HHS immediately.

    d. It is not required to take any action since the breach affected only one person.

139. Which of the following is considered a two-factor authentication system?

    a. User ID with a password

    b. User ID with voice scan

    c. Password and swipe card

    d. Password and PIN

140. Which of the following technologies would reduce the risk that information is not accessible during a server crash?

    a. RAID

    b. Server redundancy

    c. Storage area network

    d. Tape or disk backup

141. Under the HIPAA Privacy Rule, which of the following statements is true?

    a. An authorization must contain an expiration date or event.

    b. A consent for use and disclosure of information must be obtained from every patient.

    c. An authorization must be obtained for uses and disclosures for treatment, payment, and operations.

    d. A notice of privacy practices must give 10 examples of a use or disclosure for healthcare operations.

142. Which of the following security controls are built into a computer software program?

    a. Physical safeguards

    b. Administration safeguards

    c. Application safeguards

    d. Media safeguards

143. An audit log is an example of:

    a. Metadata

    b. Encryption

    c. Admissibility

    d. Data integrity

144. An HIT using her password can access and change data in the hospital's master patient index. A billing clerk, using his password, cannot perform the same function. Limiting the class of information and functions that can be performed by these two employees is managed by:

    a. Network controls

    b. Audit trails

    c. Administrative controls

    d. Access controls

145. Which of the following is an organization's planned response to protect its information in the case of a natural disaster?

    a. Administrative controls

    b. Contingency plan

    c. Audit trail

    d. Physical controls

146. Under HIPAA, which of the following is *not* named as a covered entity?

    a. Attending physician

    b. Healthcare clearinghouse

    c. Health plan

    d. Outsourced transcription company

147. Which of the following is true of the HIPAA Privacy Rule?

    a. It protects only medical information that is not already specifically protected by state law.

    b. It supersedes all state laws that conflict with it.

    c. It is federal common law.

    d. It sets a minimum (floor) of privacy requirements.

148. Which of the following is *not* an element that makes information PHI under the HIPAA Privacy Rule?

    a. Identifies an individual

    b. In the custody of or transmitted by a CE or its BA

    c. Contained within a personnel file

    d. Relates to one's health condition

149. Which of the following is a software program that tracks every access to data in the computer system?

    a. Access control

    b. Audit trail

    c. Edit check

    d. Risk assessment

150. Central City Clinic has requested that Midtown Hospital send its hospital records for Susan Hall's most recent admission to the clinic for her follow-up appointment. Which of the following statements is true?

    a. The privacy rule requires that Susan Hall complete a written authorization.

    b. The hospital may send only the discharge summary, history and physical, and operative report.

    c. The privacy rule's minimum necessary requirement does not apply.

    d. This "public interest and benefit" disclosure does not require the patient's authorization.

151. Stacy is completing her required high school community service hours by serving as a volunteer at the local hospital. In this capacity, Stacy is a(n):

    a. Business associate

    b. Covered entity

    c. Employee

    d. Workforce member

152. Lakeside Hospital has a contract with Ready-Clean, a local company, to come into the hospital to pick up all of the facility's linens for off-site laundering. Ready-Clean is:

    a. A business associate because Lane Hospital has a contract with it

    b. Not a business associate because it is a local company

    c. A business associate because its employees may see PHI

    d. Not a business associate because it does not use or disclose individually identifiable health information

153. For HIPAA implementation specifications that are addressable, which of the following statements is true?

    a. The covered entity must implement the specification.

    b. The covered entity may choose not to implement the specification if implementation is too costly.

    c. The covered entity must conduct a risk assessment to determine whether the specification is appropriate to its environment.

    d. If the covered entity is a small hospital, the specification does not have to be implemented.

154. A competent individual has the following rights concerning his or her healthcare:

    a. Right to consent to treatment and the right to destroy their original health record

    b. Right to destroy their original health record and the right to refuse treatment

    c. Right to access his or her own PHI and the right to take the original record with them

    d. Right to consent to treatment and the right to access his or her own PHI

155. Covered entities must do which of the following to comply with HIPAA security provisions?

    a. Appoint an individual who has the title of chief security officer who is responsible for security management.

    b. Conduct employee security training sessions every six months for all employees.

    c. Establish a contingency plan.

    d. Conduct technical and nontechnical evaluations every six years.

156. The health record of Kathy Smith, the plaintiff, has been subpoenaed for a deposition. The plaintiff's attorney wishes to use the records as evidence to prove his client's case. In this situation, although the record constitutes hearsay, it may be used as evidence based on the:

    a. Admissibility exception

    b. Discovery exception

    c. Direct evidence exception

    d. Business records exception

157. Jeremy Lykins was required to undergo a physical exam prior to becoming employed by San Fernando Hospital. Jeremy's medical information is:

    a. Protected by the privacy rule because it is individually identifiable

    b. Not protected by the privacy rule because it is part of a personnel record

    c. Protected by the privacy rule because it contains his physical exam results

    d. Protected by the privacy rule because it is in the custody of a covered entity

158. Burning, shredding, pulping, and pulverizing are *all* acceptable methods in which process?

    a. Deidentification of electronic documents

    b. Destruction of paper-based health records

    c. Deidentification of records stored on microfilm

    d. Destruction of electronic documents

159. The HIPAA Privacy Rule requires that covered entities must limit use, access, and disclosure of PHI to only the amount needed to accomplish the intended purpose. What concept is this an example of?

    a. Minimum necessary

    b. Notice of privacy practices

    c. Authorization

    d. Consent

160. To comply with HIPAA regulations, a hospital would make its membership in an HIE known to its patients through which of the following?

    a. Press release

    b. Notice of privacy practices

    c. Consent form

    d. Website notice

161. Which of the following statements is *not* true about a business associate agreement?

    a. It prohibits the business associate from using or disclosing PHI for any purpose other than that described in the contract with the covered entity.

    b. It allows the business associate to maintain PHI indefinitely.

    c. It prohibits the business associate from using or disclosing PHI in any way that would violate the HIPAA Privacy Rule.

    d. It requires the business associate to make available all of its books and records relating to PHI use and disclosure to the Department of Health and Human Services or its agents.

162. If a patient wants to amend his or her health record, the covered entity may require the individual to:

    a. Make an amendment request in writing and provide a rationale for the amendment.

    b. Ask the attending physician for his or her permission to amend their record.

    c. Require the patient to wait 30 days before their request will be considered and processed.

    d. Provide a court order requesting the amendment.

163. For which of the following is the custodian of health records *not* responsible?

    a. Authorized to certify records

    b. Supervising inspection and copying of records

    c. Testifying to the authenticity of records

    d. Testifying regarding the care of the patient

164. When served with a court order directing the release of health records, an individual:

    a. May ignore it

    b. Must comply with it

    c. Must request patient authorization before disclosing the records

    d. May determine whether or not to comply with it

165. The process of releasing health record documentation originally created by a different provider is called:

    a. Privileged communication

    b. Subpoena

    c. Jurisdiction

    d. Redisclosure

166. Which of the following is *not* true of notices of privacy practices?

    a. They must be made available at the site where the individual is treated.

    b. They must be posted in a prominent place.

    c. They must contain content that may not be changed.

    d. They must be prominently posted on the covered entity's website when the entity has one.

167. To comply with HIPAA, under usual circumstances, a covered entity must act on a patient's request to review or copy his or her health information within _____ days.

    a. 10

    b. 20

    c. 30

    d. 60

168. Jennifer's widowed mother is elderly and often confused. She has asked Jennifer to accompany her to the physician office visits because she often forgets to tell the physician vital information. Under the HIPAA Privacy Rule, the release of her mother's PHI to Jennifer is:

    a. Never allowed

    b. Allowed when the information is directly relevant to Jennifer's involvement in her mother's care or treatment

    c. Allowed only if Jennifer's mother is declared incompetent by a court of law

    d. Any family member is always allowed access to PHI

169. Which of the following statements is *false* with regard to the HIPAA Privacy Rule?

    a. A notice of privacy practices must be written in plain language.

    b. A notice of privacy practices must have a statement that other uses and disclosures will be made only with the individual's written authorization and that the individual may revoke such authorization.

    c. An authorization must be obtained for uses and disclosures for treatment, payment, and operations.

    d. A notice of privacy practices must give an example of a use or disclosure for healthcare operations.

170. Who owns the health record?

    a. Patient

    b. Provider who generated the information

    c. Insurance company who paid for the care recorded in the record

    d. No one

171. What is the legal term used to define the protection of health information in a patient-provider relationship?

    a. Access

    b. Confidentiality

    c. Privacy

    d. Security

172. Under HIPAA regulations, how many days does a covered entity have to respond to an individual's request for access to his or her PHI when the PHI is stored off-site?

    a. 10 days beyond the original requirement

    b. 30 days

    c. 60 days

    d. 90 days

173. Written business associate agreements are required with:

    a. Every company where work is outsourced

    b. Any outside company that handles electronic data

    c. Every outside company

    d. Any outside company that handles electronic PHI

174. Which of the following is an example of a business associate?

    a. Contract coding professional

    b. Environmental services department

    c. Hospital security officer

    d. Employee with access to e-PHI

175. What type of health record policy dictates how long individual health records must remain available for authorized use?

    a. Disclosure policies

    b. Legal policies

    c. Retention policies

    d. Redisclosure policies

176. Which document directs an individual to bring originals or copies of records to court?

    a. Summons

    b. Subpoena *ad testificandum*

    c. Subpoena *duces tecum*

    d. Deposition

177. Which of the following statements about the directory of patients maintained by a covered entity is true?

    a. Individuals must be given an opportunity to restrict or deny permission to place information about them in the directory.

    b. Individuals must provide a written authorization before information about them can be placed in the directory.

    c. The directory may contain only identifying information such as the patient's name and birth date.

    d. The directory may contain private information as long as it is kept confidential.

178. Which of the following is *not* true about the notice of privacy practices?

    a. It must include a description of the patient's right to amend PHI.

    b. It must include a description of the right to request restrictions on certain uses and disclosures.

    c. It must explain the patient's right to inspect and copy PHI.

    d. It must include at least two examples of how information is used for both treatment and operations.

179. Which of the following defines the legal health record (LHR)?

    a. A defined subset of all patient-specific data created or accumulated by a healthcare provider that may be released to third parties in response to a legally permissible request for patient information.

    b. An entire set of information created or accumulated by a healthcare provider that may be released to third parties in response to a legally permissible request for patient information.

    c. A set of patient-specific data created or accumulated by a healthcare provider that is defined to be legal by the local, state, or federal authorities.

    d. A set of patient-specific data that is defined to be legal by state or federal statute and that is legally permissible to provide in response to requests for patient information.

180. Which of the following is the legal term used to describe when a patient has the right to maintain control over certain personal information?

    a. Access

    b. Confidentiality

    c. Privacy

    d. Security

181. Which of the following has access to personally identifiable data without authorization or subpoena?

    a. Insurance company for life insurance eligibility

    b. Public health department for disease reporting purposes

    c. The patient's attorney

    d. Workers' compensation for disability claim settlement

182. Community Hospital is discussing restricting the access that physicians have to electronic health records. The medical record committee is divided on how to approach this issue. Some committee members maintain that all information should be available, whereas others maintain that HIPAA restricts access. The HIM director is part of the committee. Which of the following should the director advise the committee?

    a. HIPAA restricts the access of physicians to all information.

    b. The minimum necessary concept does not apply to disclosures made for treatment purposes; therefore, physician access should not be restricted.

    c. The minimum necessary concept does not apply to disclosures made for treatment purposes, but the organization must define what physicians need as part of their treatment role.

    d. The minimum necessary concept applies only to attending physicians and, therefore, restriction of access must be implemented.

183. When a patient revokes authorization for release of information after a healthcare facility has already released the information, the facility in this case:

    a. May be prosecuted for invasion of privacy

    b. Has become subject to civil action

    c. Has violated the security regulations of HIPAA

    d. Is protected by the Privacy Act

184. Mrs. Bolton is an angry patient who resents her physicians "bossing her around." She refuses to take a portion of the medications the nurses bring to her pursuant to physician orders and is verbally abusive to the patient care assistants. Of the following options, the most appropriate way to document Mrs. Bolton's behavior in the patient medical record is:

    a. Mean

    b. Noncompliant and hostile toward staff

    c. Belligerent and out of line

    d. A pain in the neck

185. As the corporate director of HIM services and enterprise privacy officer, you are asked to review a patient's health record in preparation for a legal proceeding for a malpractice case. The lawsuit was brought by the patient 72 days after the procedure. The health record contains a summary of two procedures that were dictated 95 days after the procedure. The physician in question has a longstanding history of being lackadaisical with record completion practices. Previous concerns regarding this physician's record maintenance practices had been reported to the facility's Credentialing Committee. Is this information about the physician's record maintenance practices admissible in court?

    a. This information could be rejected because the physician dictated the procedure note after the malpractice suit was filed.

    b. This information will be admissible in court because it is part of the patient's health record.

    c. This information could be rejected because it is not relevant to the malpractice case.

    d. This information will be rejected because the patient did not authorize its release.

186. The sister of a patient requests the HIM department to release copies of her brother's health record to her. She states that because the physician documented her name as her brother's caregiver that HIPAA regulations apply and that she may receive copies of her brother's health record. In this case, how should the HIM department proceed?

    a. Provide the copies as requested since the sister was a caregiver.

    b. Provide only copies of the reports where the sister's name is mentioned.

    c. Refuse the request.

    d. Refer the individual to legal counsel.

187. The Health Insurance Portability and Accountability Act (HIPAA):

    a. Applies to anyone who collects health information

    b. Preempts all state laws

    c. Provides a federal floor for healthcare privacy

    d. Duplicates the Joint Commission standards

188. Protection of healthcare information from damage, loss, and unauthorized alteration is also known as:

    a. Data accuracy

    b. Privacy

    c. Results management

    d. Data security

189. Which of the following would *not* be considered a HIPAA data breach?

    a. Release of employee salary data

    b. Lost laptop that contains patient names, addresses, and ICD codes

    c. The use of a patient's name and social security number by an employee to get a credit card

    d. Unauthorized use of PHI by a hospital employee

190. In regard to data security, what is the purpose of a red flag?

    a. Elevate security protection levels

    b. Increase audit trail reporting

    c. Raise concerns over security awareness

    d. Sound an alert to a potential identify theft

191. Recently, a state senator was admitted to your facility for a serious medical condition. The facility privacy officer has been tasked with reviewing access logs daily to determine which of the following?

    a. Whether or not the patient is fit to continue public service

    b. What information should be shared with the media

    c. That the patient has received adequate care

    d. Whether all access by hospital employees was appropriate

192. The HIM manager at Community Hospital is responsible for reviewing audit trails detailing potential access issues within the EHR. Which one of the following would be a type of activity that the manager would want to review?

   a. Every access to every data element or document type that occurred within the facility

   b. Whether the person viewed, created, updated, or deleted information belonging to a patient with the same last name

   c. Physical location of the redundant servers used for backup

   d. Whether all patients setup accounts in the patient portal

193. Community Hospital is identifying strategies to minimize the security risks associated with employees leaving their workstations unattended. Which of the following solutions will minimize the security risk of unattended workstations?

   a. Use biometrics for access to the system.

   b. Implement firewall and virus protection.

   c. Implement automatic session terminations.

   d. Install encryption and similar devices.

194. A notice that suspends the process or destruction of health records is called a:

   a. Subpoena

   b. Consent form

   c. Rule

   d. Legal hold

195. A physician takes the medical records of a group of HIV-positive patients out of the hospital to complete research tasks at home. The physician mistakenly leaves the records in a restaurant, where they are read by a newspaper reporter who publishes an article that identifies the patients. The physician can be sued for:

   a. Slander

   b. Willful infliction of mental distress

   c. Libel

   d. Invasion of privacy

196. A visitor to the hospital looks at the screen of the admitting clerk's computer workstation when she leaves her desk to copy some admitting documents. What security mechanism would best have minimized this security breach?

   a. Document controls

   b. Audit controls

   c. Automatic log-off controls

   d. Device and media controls

197. A laboratory employee forgot his password to the computer system while trying to record the results for a STAT request. He asked his coworker to log in for him so that he could record the results and said he would then contact technical support to reset his password. What controls should have been in place to minimize this security breach?

    a. Access controls

    b. Security incident procedures

    c. Security management process

    d. Workforce security awareness training

198. Proud grandparents of a new baby born at Riverview Hospital directly submitted an announcement with the birth information directly to the local newspaper. The local newspaper printed the information about the birth, should the newspaper be concerned about the HIPAA Privacy Rule?

    a. No, because the newspaper is not bound by HIPAA.

    b. No, because the birth information is never PHI.

    c. Yes, because the newspaper is a covered entity under HIPAA.

    d. Yes, because the birth information was submitted directly by the hospital.

199. A valid authorization requires a(n):

    a. Statement that a notice of privacy practices has been provided

    b. Expiration date or event

    c. Statement that patient understands their rights related to PHI

    d. Patient account number

200. When can a covered entity deny an individual's request to restrict the use or disclosure of his or her PHI?

    a. Never

    b. In all cases

    c. In all cases, except for disclosures to a health plan where the individual has paid for a service or item completely out of pocket

    d. In all cases, except for disclosures where the patient has requested the restriction in writing

201. A funeral home is contacted to retrieve a patient's body. This contact and disclosure of information about the decedent is:

    a. A public interest and benefit exception to the authorization requirement

    b. Only permissible if the decedent's next of kin has given written authorization for information about the decedent to be disclosed to the funeral home

    c. A violation of the HIPAA Privacy Rule

    d. Subject to a HIPAA consent by the next of kin

202. A nurse called Katie by her first name in a physician's office when Katie was to be seen by the physician. This was:

    a. An incidental disclosure

    b. Not subject to the minimum necessary requirement

    c. A disclosure for payment purposes

    d. An automatic violation of the privacy rule

203. Mary Jane accesses the health insurance policy numbers of patients for billing purposes. This activity best exemplifies:

    a. Ownership and control

    b. Disclosure

    c. Request for information

    d. Use

204. Which of the following individual's medical information is no longer protected by the HIPAA Privacy Rule?

    a. Roxanne, who has been deceased 5 years

    b. Carrie, who has been deceased 10 years

    c. Ray, who has been deceased 25 years

    d. Charles, who has been deceased 75 years

205. A notice of privacy practices should include a statement:

    a. Explaining that individuals may complain to the Secretary of HHS if they believe that their privacy rights have been violated

    b. That parents may access the PHI of their minor children

    c. That state law may not be preempted by HIPAA

    d. That the HIPAA Privacy Rule pertains only to healthcare providers

206. Citizen State Bank offered a flu shot clinic to its employees that are covered under the employee health plan. The employee health plan administered and tracked the flu shots in their own records. In this situation, would HIPAA rules apply for Citizen State Bank?

    a. No, because bank employees did not administer the flu shots.

    b. Yes, because Citizen State Bank would be considered a covered entity under HIPAA.

    c. No, because Citizen State Bank is not considered a covered entity under HIPAA.

    d. Yes, because their employee health plan administered the shots.

Domain 3 *Data Analytics and Use*

207. Given the numbers 47, 20, 11, 33, 30, 30, 35, and 50, what is the mode?

    a. 30

    b. 32

    c. 32.5

    d. 35

208. Community Memorial Hospital had 25 inpatient deaths, including newborns, during the month of June. The hospital had a total of 500 discharges for the same period, including deaths of adults, children, and newborns. The hospital's gross death rate for the month of June was:

    a. 0.05%

    b. 2%

    c. 5%

    d. 20%

209. The HIM data analytics professional is reviewing a chart (shown here) on nosocomial infections presented by the hospital's infection control committee. The committee is reporting that the decrease in infection rate has accelerated during the past 10 years. What comments should the data analytics professional make?

    a. Concur with the conclusion of the committee

    b. State that the greatest decrease in infection rate in a year took place in 2005

    c. State that the greatest decrease in infection rate occurred in 1960 and 1970

    d. Request a new data chart be presented that accurately reflects the trend of infection rate

210. City Hospital's HIM department made a decision to discontinue outsourcing its release of information (ROI) function and perform the function in house. Because of HIPAA implementation, the department wanted better control over tracking release of information. Given the graph shown here, how would you evaluate the ROI revenue growth?

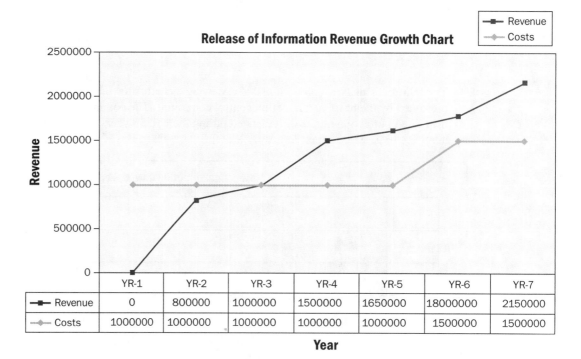

Release of Information Revenue Growth Chart

	YR-1	YR-2	YR-3	YR-4	YR-5	YR-6	YR-7
Revenue	0	800000	1000000	1500000	1650000	18000000	2150000
Costs	1000000	1000000	1000000	1000000	1000000	1500000	1500000

Year

   a. The ROI function continues to cost more than revenue generated.

   b. Annualized revenue for YR-7 is more than the costs.

   c. The ROI function costs are inversely related to revenue generated.

   d. The ROI costs for YR-7 are greater than the revenue.

211. After the types of cases to be included in a trauma registry have been determined, what is the next step in data acquisition?

   a. Registering

   b. Defining

   c. Abstracting

   d. Case finding

212. One of the pediatricians at Community Physician's Clinic worked with a software vendor to get a display of the patients she currently has in the hospital on her smartphone that lets her know current information such as lab results, vital signs, medications given. This describes which of the following?

   a. Big data

   b. Descriptive analytics screen

   c. Dashboard

   d. Descriptive tablet

213. The business office at Community Hospital is looking at software that can help with decreasing their fraud and abuse cases. The software claims to be able to flag those patients who would most likely be involved in fraud by examining many databases at the same time and finding those patients with demographic discrepancies. This is an example of:

    a. Descriptive analytics

    b. Predictive analytics

    c. Inferential statistics

    d. Descriptive statistics

214. Community Hospital discharged nine patients on April 1. The length of stay for each of the patients was as follows: patient A, 1 day; patient B, 5 days; patient C, 3 days; patient D, 3 days; patient E, 8 days; patient F, 8 days; patient G, 8 days; patient H, 9 days; patient I, 9 days. What was the median length of stay?

    a. Five days

    b. Six days

    c. Eight days

    d. Nine days

215. At Community Hospital, each full-time employee is required to work 2,080 hours annually. The following table shows the amount of time that four employees were absent from work over the past year.

Community Hospital Health Information Management Department Coding Section Absentee Report Annual Statistics, 20XX		
Employee Name	**Vacation Hours Used**	**Sick Leave Hours Used**
A	40	6
B	22	16
C	36	8
D	80	32

Which employee had the highest absentee rate?

    a. Employee A

    b. Employee B

    c. Employee C

    d. Employee D

216. The following data were derived from a comparative discharge database for hip and femur procedures:

Comparative Data on Hip and Femur Procedures for Current Year				
	Hospital A	Hospital B	Hospital C	Hospital D
Hip procedures	2,300	1,467	2,567	1,100
Femur procedures	988	1,245	1,067	678

These data can best be described as:

a. Aggregate

b. Identifiable

c. Patient specific

d. Primary

217. In a frequency distribution, the lowest value is 5, and the highest value is 20. What is the range?

a. 5 to 20

b. 7.5

c. 15

d. 20 to 5

218. What is the mean for the following frequency distribution: 10, 15, 20, 25, 25?

a. 19

b. 20

c. 47.5

d. 95

219. Which of the following is a format problem in this table?

Sex	Number	Percentage
Male	3,000	37.5%
Female	5,000	62.5%
Unknown	6,500	73.6%
Total	8,000	100%

a. The title is missing.

b. Variable names are missing.

c. There are blank cells.

d. Row totals are inaccurate.

220. Mr. Jones was admitted to the hospital on March 21 and discharged on April 1. What was the length of stay for Mr. Jones?

    a. 5 days

    b. 10 days

    c. 11 days

    d. 15 days

221. Which of the following is an example of how an internal user utilizes secondary data?

    a. State infectious disease reporting

    b. Birth certificates

    c. Death certificates

    d. Benchmarking with other facilities

222. Community Hospital had 25 inpatient deaths, including newborns, for the month of June. The hospital performed five autopsies for the same period. What was the gross autopsy rate for the hospital for June?

    a. 0.02%

    b. 5%

    c. 20%

    d. 200%

223. If you want to display the parts of a whole in graphic form, what graphic technique would you use?

    a. Table

    b. Histogram

    c. Line graph

    d. Pie chart

224. Which term is used to describe the number of inpatients present at the census-taking time each day plus the number of inpatients who were both admitted and discharged after the census-taking time the previous day?

    a. Inpatient bed occupancy rate

    b. Bed count

    c. Average daily census

    d. Daily inpatient census

225. Suppose that five patients stayed in the hospital for a total of 27 days. Which term would be used to describe the result of the calculation 27 divided by 5?

    a. Average length of stay

    b. Total length of stay

    c. Patient length of stay

    d. Average patient census

226. Which rate is used to compare the number of inpatient deaths to the total number of inpatient deaths and discharges?

    a. Net hospital death rate

    b. Maternal hospital death rate

    c. Gross death rate

    d. Adjusted hospital death rate

227. Which unit of measure is used to indicate the services received by one inpatient in a 24-hour period?

    a. Inpatient service day

    b. Volume of services

    c. Average occupancy charges

    d. Length of services provided

228. What term is used for the number of inpatients present at any one time in a healthcare facility?

    a. Average daily census

    b. Census

    c. Inpatient service day

    d. Length of stay

229. Which rate describes the probability or risk of illness in a population over a period of time?

    a. Mortality

    b. Prevalence

    c. Incidence

    d. Morbidity

230. A statewide database is used by your performance improvement department each month to compare other facilities' readmission rates to your facility's rates. This is an example of:

    a. Internal data

    b. External data

    c. Ratio data

    d. Nominal data

231. Why is the MEDPAR file limited in terms of being used for research purposes?

    a. It only contains Medicare patients.

    b. It only provides demographic data about patients.

    c. It uses diagnoses and procedure codes.

    d. It breaks charges down by specific types of service.

232. At Community Hospital, each full-time employee is required to work 2,080 hours annually. The following table displays the amount of time that five employees were absent from work over the past year.

Community Hospital Health Information Management Department Coding Section Absentee Report Annual Statistics, 20XX		
Employee Name	Vacation Hours Used	Sick Leave Hours Used
A	40	6
B	22	16
C	36	8
D	80	32
E	16	40

What is the total sick leave rate for this group of employees for the year?

a. 0.29%

b. 0.98%

c. 1.29%

d. 1.54%

233. Use the information provided to determine which of the following statements is correct?

MS-DRG	MDC	Type	MS-DRG Title	Weight	Discharges	Geometric Mean	Arithmetic Mean
191	04	MED	Chronic obstructive pulmonary disease w CC	0.8843	10	2.9	3.5
192	04	MED	Chronic obstructive pulmonary disease w/o CC/MCC	0.6956	20	2.4	2.8
193	04	MED	Simple pneumonia & pleurisy w MCC	1.3120	10	4.1	5.1
194	04	MED	Simple pneumonia & pleurisy w CC	0.8639	20	3.1	3.7
195	04	MED	Simple pneumonia & pleurisy w/o CC/MCC	0.6658	10	2.5	2.9

a. In each MS-DRG, the geometric mean is lower than the arithmetic mean.

b. In each MS-DRG, the arithmetic mean is lower than the geometric mean.

c. The higher the number of patients in each MS-DRG, the greater the geometric mean for that MS-DRG.

d. The geometric means are lower in MS-DRGs that are associated with a CC or MCC.

234. Given the following information, in which city is the GPCI the highest for practice expense?

City	Work GPCI	Practice Expense GPCI	Malpractice Expense GPCI
Sample Geographical Practice Cost Indices (GPCI) for Selected Cities			
St. Louis	1.000	0.968	1.064
Dallas	1.009	1.001	0.969
Seattle	1.020	1.098	0.785
Philadelphia	1.015	1.084	1.619

a. St. Louis

b. Dallas

c. Seattle

d. Philadelphia

235. Which term is used to describe the number of calendar days that a patient is hospitalized?

a. Average length of stay

b. Length of stay

c. Occupancy rate

d. Level of service

236. Which of the following is the unique identifier in the relational database patient table?

Patient #	Patient Last Name	Patient First Name	Date of Birth
Patient Table			
021234	Smith	Donna	03/21/1944
022366	Jones	Donna	04/09/1960
034457	Smith	Mary	08/21/1977

a. Patient last name

b. Patient last and first name

c. Patient date of birth

d. Patient number

237. The Medical Staff Executive Committee has requested a report that identifies all medical staff members who have been suspended in the past six months due to delinquent health records. This is an example of what type of report?

a. Ad hoc or demand

b. Annual report

c. Exception

d. Periodic scheduled

238. Hospital A discharges 10,000 patients per year. Hospital B is located in the same town and discharges 5,000 patients per year. At Hospital B's medical staff committee meeting, a physician reports that he is concerned about the quality of care at Hospital B because the hospital has double the number of deaths per year than Hospital A. The HIM director is attending the meeting in a staff position. Which of the following actions should the director take?

    a. Make no comment since this is a medical staff meeting.

    b. Agree with the physician that the data suggest a quality issue.

    c. Suggest that the data be adjusted for possible differences in type and volume of patients treated.

    d. Suggest that an audit be done immediately to determine the cause of deaths within the hospital.

239. Community Hospital has compared its admission-type patient-profile data for two consecutive years. From a performance improvement standpoint, which admission types should the hospital examine for possible changes in capacity handling?

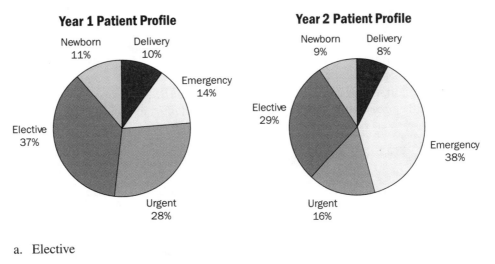

    a. Elective

    b. Emergency

    c. Newborn

    d. Urgent

240. A report that lists the ICD-10-CM codes associated with each physician in a healthcare facility can be used to assess the quality of the physician's services before he or she is:

    a. Scheduled for a coding audit

    b. Subjected to corrective action

    c. Recommended for staff reappointment

    d. Involved in an in-house training program

241. The following table compares Community Hospital's pneumonia length of stay (observed LOS) to the pneumonia LOS of similar hospitals (expected LOS). Given this data, where might Community Hospital want to focus attention on its pneumonia LOS?

LOS Summary for Pneumonia by Clinical Specialty				
Clinical Specialty	Cases	Observed LOS	Expected LOS	Savings Opportunity
Cardiology	1	6	6.36	0
Family Practice	17	8.47	6.26	38
Internal Medicine	34	3.82	4.89	−36
Endocrinology	1	3	3.93	−1
Pediatrics	7	3.43	3.55	−1

a. Cardiology

b. Endocrinology

c. Family practice

d. Internal medicine

242. The following data has been collected about the HIM department's coding productivity as part of the organization's total quality improvement program. Which of the following is the best assessment of this data?

Coder	Work Output (All Records Coded)	Total Hours Worked	Average Work Output per Hour	Completed Work Percentage	Completed Work Output (Records Coded Accurately)	Completed Work per Hour Worked
A	500	140 (full time)	3.57	91%	455	3.25
B	475	140 (full time)	3.39	96%	456	3.26
C	300	80 (part time)	3.75	85%	240	3.00
D	350	80 (part time)	4.69	70%	245	3.06
Department Average			3.69			3.17

> **Work Output:** Number of work units as recorded by the employee or the process
>
> **Total Hours Worked:** Number of hours worked by the employee to produce work, which does not include time on meals, breaks, and meetings
>
> **Average Work Output per Hour:** Work output divided by total hours worked
>
> **Completed Work Percentage:** Percentage of records coded accurately
>
> **Completed Work Output:** Work output multiplied by completed work percentage
>
> **Completed Work per Hour Worked:** Completed work output divided by total hours worked

a. Part-time coding professionals are more productive than full-time coding professionals.

b. Full-time coding professionals are more productive than part-time coding professionals.

c. All coding professionals produce more than the departmental average.

d. Part-time coding professionals exceed the departmental average.

243. Community Hospital performed a cost-savings analysis between its current on-site coding processes and an e-WebCoding telecommuting model. What does the cost analysis show in the following graph?

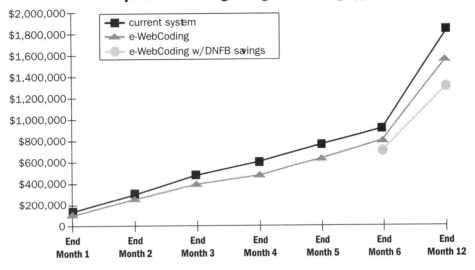

Projected Cost Savings Using e-WebCoding Application

a. The current system saves more than the e-WebCoding system would.

b. The current system reduces DNFB significantly.

c. Cost comparison reflects a net reduction in overall expenses on a monthly basis for the e-WebCoding system.

d. There is not enough information to make a determination.

244. Given the following information, from which payer does the hospital proportionately receive the least amount of payment?

Payer	Charges	Payments	Adjustments	Charges	Payments	Adjustments
BC/BS	$450,000	$360,000	$90,000	23%	31%	12%
Commercial	$250,000	$200,000	$50,000	13%	17%	6%
Medicaid	$350,000	$75,000	$275,000	18%	6%	36%
Medicare	$750,000	$495,000	$255,000	39%	42%	33%
TRICARE	$150,000	$50,000	$100,000	7%	4%	13%
Total	$1,950,000	$1,180,000	$770,000	100%	100%	100%

a. BC/BS

b. TRICARE

c. Medicare

d. Medicaid

245. Which of the following is made up of claims data from Medicare claims submitted by acute-care hospitals and skilled nursing facilities?

a. NPDB

b. MEDPAR

c. HIPDB

d. UHDDS

246. Which autopsy rate compares the number of autopsies performed on hospital inpatients to the total number of inpatient deaths for the same period of time?

    a. Net

    b. Gross

    c. Hospital

    d. Average

247. What do the wedges or divisions in a pie graph represent?

    a. Frequency groups

    b. Various data

    c. Percentages

    d. Classes

248. Within the context of the inpatient prospective payment system, how is the case-mix index calculated?

    a. The sum of all relative weights divided by the total number of discharges

    b. The total number of inpatient service days divided by the total number of discharges

    c. The sum of all MDCs divided by the total number of discharges

    d. The total number of inpatient beds divided by the total number of discharges

249. Using the information in the following table, calculate the C-section rate at University Hospital for the semiannual period.

University Hospital Obstetrics Service Semiannual Statistics July-December, 20XX	
Admissions	672
Discharges and Deaths:	
Delivered	504
Not Delivered	147
Aborted	21
Vaginal deliveries	403
C-sections	101

    a. 15.03%

    b. 19.24%

    c. 20.04%

    d. 25.06%

250. Your administrator has asked you to generate a report that gives the number of hypertension patients last year. This is an example of:

    a. Descriptive analytics

    b. Predictive analytics

    c. Prescriptive analytics

    d. Real-time analysis

251. Community Hospital is using a system that will help them detect when intracranial pressure becomes high in patients with a recent CVA that will quickly send an alert to the physician. This is an example of:

    a. Descriptive analytics

    b. Predictive analytics

    c. Prescriptive analytics

    d. Real-time analysis

252. In the community clinic Dr. Simpson, an interventional cardiologist, saw 270 patients last quarter. Of those, he performed stent procedures on 182 patients and angioplasty procedures on 88 patients. What is the proportion of Dr. Simpson's patients who have had stent procedures?

    a. 0.67

    b. 0.45

    c. 0.33

    d. Unable to determine

253. Which of the following reportable diseases usually requires reporting within 24 hours of a suspected diagnosis?

    a. Chicken pox

    b. Mumps

    c. Measles

    d. Pertussis

254. The type of statistics that makes a best guess about a larger group of data by drawing conclusions from a smaller group of data is called:

    a. Descriptive statistics

    b. Inferential statistics

    c. Generalized statistics

    d. Mathematical statistics

255. A managed care organization is using a system that examines the past healthcare behaviors of their patients to determine their future costs for their healthcare. This is an example of:

    a. Descriptive analytics

    b. Predictive modeling

    c. Prescriptive analytics

    d. Real-time analysis

256. A secondary data source includes which of the following?

    a. Vital statistics

    b. The medical record

    c. The physician's index

    d. A videotape of a counseling session

257. What is the official count of inpatients taken at midnight called?

   a. Average daily census

   b. Census

   c. Daily inpatient census

   d. Inpatient service days

258. In the relational database shown here, the patient table and the visit table are related by which of the following?

Patient Table			
Patient #	**Patient Last Name**	**Patient First Name**	**Date of Birth**
021234	Smith	Donna	03/21/1944
022366	Jones	William	04/09/1960
034457	Collins	Mary	08/21/1977

Visit Table			
Visit #	**Date of Visit**	**Practitioner #**	**Patient #**
0045678	11/12/2021	456	021234
0045679	11/12/2021	997	021234
0045680	11/12/2021	456	034457

   a. Visit number

   b. Date of visit

   c. Patient number

   d. Practitioner number

259. Case finding is a method used to:

   a. Identify patients who have been seen or treated in a facility for a particular disease or condition for inclusion in a registry

   b. Define which cases are to be included in a registry

   c. Identify trends and changes in the incidence of disease

   d. Identify facility-based trends

260. Data found on sites such as Medicare.gov use aggregated data to describe the experiences of unique types of patients with one or more aspects of their care. This data collection is called?

   a. Patient-specific

   b. Administrative

   c. Comparative

   d. Detailed

261. Certificates, such as those for births and fetal-deaths, are reported by hospitals to the individual state registrars and maintained permanently. State vital statistics registrars then compile the data and report them to which of the following:

   a. National Center for Health Statistics

   b. Agency for Healthcare Research and Quality

   c. Health Services Research

   d. National Statistics Research

262. The HIM professional reported to the quality improvement committee at Community Hospital that there were 58 patients with influenza discharged from the hospital in January. Of those 58 patients, 3 patients died. What is the case fatality rate for influenza for January?

    a. 1.60%

    b. 5.17%

    c. 0.10%

    d. 94.8%

263. Information that has been taken from the health records of injured patients and entered into the trauma registry database has been:

    a. Aggregated

    b. Mapped

    c. Abstracted

    d. Queried

264. The HIM department at Community Hospital has three full time coding professionals. One is considered the lead coding professional and his salary is $20.35 per hour. One coding professional is a new graduate who makes $15.50 per hour and the third coding professional is an experienced employee who earns $18.90 per hour. The lead coding professional codes four records per hour; the new coding professional codes three records per hour and their experienced coding professional codes six records per hour. Using a 7.5-hour productive day, what is the unit cost for the lead coder?

    a. $3.36 per record

    b. $4.49 per record

    c. $5.43 per record

    d. $5.51 per record

265. Analyze the following report of physician deficiency rates and determine which physician has the lowest deficiency rate for H&Ps completed within 24 hours of admission.

Community Hospital Health Information Services Physician Documentation Deficiencies January 20XX			
Physician No.	No. Admissions	No. of H&Ps Not Completed within 24 Hours of Admission	Rate of Deficiency
102	189	5	2.64
237	234	4	1.71
391	98	8	8.16
518	122	5	4.10
637	178	3	1.69

    a. 102

    b. 237

    c. 391

    d. 637

266. Suppose that 6 males and 14 females are in a class of 20 students with the data reported as 3/1. What term could be used to describe the comparison?

    a. Average

    b. Percentage

    c. Proportion

    d. Rate

267. One of the questions on the patient satisfaction survey that is sent to the patient after discharge asks for the number of times the nurses checked the patient's vital signs in a day. This is an example of which type of data?

    a. Qualitative

    b. Interval

    c. Nominal

    d. Quantitative

268. The Information Services Department has requested information about the electronic signature system being used in your facility. They would like to know the locations where physicians are accessing the system. Review the information in the following table and determine which site has the highest percentage of use.

Community Hospital Electronic Signature System 500 Physicians on Staff; 489 Using the System		
Site	No. of Physicians Using the System at This Site	% of Physicians Using the System at This Site
Medicine, 2 West	54	11.04%
Medicine, 2 East	62	12.68%
Pediatrics, 3 West	42	8.59%
Obstetrics, 1 West	12	2.45%
Physician's lounge	87	17.79%
HIM department	65	13.29%
Personal mobile device	92	18.81%
Physician home	75	15.34%

    a. HIM department

    b. Obstetrics, 1 West

    c. Personal mobile device

    d. Physician home

269. A celebrity injured while on vacation was admitted to the local community hospital for treatment of a fracture. On day two of the admission, the hospital was contacted by several media agencies stating that they were aware the patient was at the facility and requesting information about the current medical condition of this high profile celebrity patient. The CEO is concerned that an employee has shared information to the media regarding this patient. The facility privacy officer was tasked with determining if a facility employee leaked this information to the press. How would the privacy officer begin this analysis?

    a. Create a new policy about high-profile patient privacy.

    b. Start by discussing the situation with the media to resolve their inquiries.

    c. Contact employees in the facility.

    d. Review audit trail information to determine which employees have accessed this patient's information.

270. A family practitioner in your local physician's clinic saw 150 adults in one week for their annual physical examinations. Sixty-seven received the flu vaccine and three patients received the pneumococcal pneumonia vaccine. What is the rate of the flu vaccine administration for this physician?

    a. 44.7%

    b. 67.0%

    c. 20.0%

    d. 447%

271. Which of the following is used to plot the points for two variables that may be related to each other in some way?

    a. Force-field analysis

    b. Pareto chart

    c. Root cause analysis

    d. Scatter diagram

272. The coding department at Community Physician's Clinic developed the following report for the denials committee at the clinic. The billing report shows the following information. Using the following information, identify which payment source has the highest denial rate.

Community Physician's Clinic Coding Department Denials – October, 20XX			
Payment Source	Number of Claims Sent	Number of Denials	Percentage of Denials
Medicare	460	43	9.35%
Medicaid	345	35	10.14%
TRICARE	182	14	7.69%
Commercial payers	1307	83	6.35%
Worker's Compensation	6	1	16.17%
Total	2300	176	7.65%

    a. Medicare

    b. Commercial payers

    c. Worker's Compensation

    d. TRICARE

273. Using the information in this table, calculate the vaginal delivery rate at University Hospital for the semiannual period.

University Hospital Obstetrics Service Semiannual Statistics July-December, 20XX	
Admissions	672
Discharges and Deaths:	
Delivered	504
Not Delivered	147
Aborted	21
Vaginal deliveries	403
C-sections	101

   a. 20.04%

   b. 59.97%

   c. 84.13%

   d. 79.96%

274. The facility privacy officer is visited at the hospital by a recent patient who is concerned that her nosy neighbor, who happens to be a hospital employee, accessed her EHR inappropriately in order to tell other neighbors about the patient's health conditions. In order to determine this occurred, the privacy officer requests an audit log of activity within the patient's health record. What part of the audit log would the privacy officer need to first analyze to determine if this patient complaint is valid?

   a. The physician documentation from her recent stay regarding the patient's health conditions

   b. Whether the patient had requested any amendments to her record

   c. If the record has any deficiencies that would cause the record to be delinquent

   d. Which employees viewed, created, updated, or deleted information

275. The coding department at Community Physician's Clinic developed the following report for the denials committee at the clinic. Use the billing report to determine how many hours it will take to reconcile these denials if each denial takes 1.5 hours to review and resubmit the bill.

Community Physician's Clinic Coding Department Denials – October, 20XX			
Payment Source	**Number of Claims Sent**	**Number of Denials**	**Percentage of Denials**
Medicare	460	43	9.35%
Medicaid	345	35	10.14%
TRICARE	182	14	7.69%
Commercial payers	1307	83	6.35%
Worker's Compensation	6	1	16.17%
Total	2300	176	7.65%

a. 11.46 hours

b. 264 hours

c. 3450 hours

d. Unable to determine

276. On October 1st, a hurricane hit a small coastal community, which has a community hospital licensed for 50 beds. Hospital staff set up 10 additional beds around the facility and used three labor room beds and two treatment room beds in order to help take care of patients. Which of the following would be the denominator used to determine the percentage of occupancy for October 1st?

a. 50

b. 60

c. 63

d. 65

277. The number of inpatients present in a healthcare facility at any given time is called a:

a. Survey

b. Census

c. Sample

d. Enumeration

278. The Information Services department has requested information about the electronic signature system being used in your facility. They would like to know the locations where physicians are accessing the system. Review the information in the table here. What is the percentage of physicians not using the electronic signature system?

Community Hospital Electronic Signature System 500 Physicians on Staff; 489 Using the System		
Site	No. of Physicians Using the System at This Site	% of Physicians Using the System at This Site
Medicine, 2 West	54	11.04%
Medicine, 2 East	62	12.68%
Pediatrics, 3 West	42	8.59%
Obstetrics, 1 West	12	2.45%
Physician's lounge	87	17.79%
HIM department	65	13.29%
Personal mobile device	92	18.81%
Physician home	75	15.34%

a. 2.2%

b. 2.45%

c. 18.81%

d. 99.99%

279. Given the following information, which of the following has the lowest work RVU?

Sample RVUs for Selected HCPCS Codes				
HCPCS Code	Description	Work RVU	Practice Expense RVU	Malpractice Expense RVU
99204	Office visit	2.43	1.20	0.23
10080	I&D of pilonidal cyst, simple	1.22	1.58	0.20
45380	Colonoscopy with biopsy	4.43	2.72	0.67
52601	TURP, complete	15.26	8.04	1.50

   a. Office visit

   b. I&D of pilonidal cyst, simple

   c. Colonoscopy with biopsy

   d. TURP, complete

280. The HIM department at Community Hospital has three full time coding professionals. One is considered the lead coding professional and his salary is $20.35 per hour. One coding professional is a new graduate who makes $15.50 per hour and the third coding professional is an experienced employee who earns $18.90 per hour. The lead coding professional codes four records per hour; the new graduate coding professional codes three records per hour and their experienced coding professional codes six records per hour. Using a 7.5-hour productive day, what is the unit cost for the new graduate coding professional?

   a. $3.36 per record

   b. $4.49 per record

   c. $5.43 per record

   d. $5.51 per record

281. Which type of analytics allows users to prescribe a number of different possible actions?

   a. Descriptive analytics

   b. Predictive analytics

   c. Prescriptive analytics

   d. Real-time analysis

282. In analyzing the reason for changes in a hospital's Medicare case-mix index over time, the analyst should start with which of the following levels of detail?

   a. Account level

   b. MS-DRG level

   c. MDC level

   d. MS-DRG triples, pairs, and singles

283. The Medical Record Committee wants to determine if the hospital is in compliance with medical staff rules and regulations for medical record delinquency rates. The HIM director has compiled a report that shows that records are delinquent for an average of 29 days after discharge. Given this information, what can the committee conclude?

   a. Delinquency rate is within medical staff rules and regulations.

   b. All physicians are performing at optimal levels.

   c. The chart deficiency process is working well.

   d. Data are insufficient to determine whether the hospital is in compliance.

284. The term used to describe breaking data elements into the level of detail needed to retrieve the data is:

    a. Normalization

    b. Data definitions

    c. Primary key

    d. Data management system

285. You have been asked by the Chief Medical Officer of Carson Hospital to research the COVID-19 pandemic in your community and its impact on the hospital. You begin with determining the average age, median length of stay, gender and race admission rates, and insurance coverage. Identify the type of data analytics performed in this scenario.

    a. Predictive analytics

    b. Diagnostic analytics

    c. Prescriptive analytics

    d. Descriptive analytics

286. The revenue cycle director of University Hospital is interested in comparing the reliability of charge capture for infusion services using computer-based coding versus using a staff member to determine the items to charge. This is an example of what type of reliability?

    a. Inter-rater reliability

    b. Internal consistency

    c. Content validity

    d. External consistency

287. Dr. Hawkins, a cardiac surgeon, had 32 patients last month who had surgery in the Surgery Service at Community Hospital. One of his patients died within 10 days of surgery. What was the postoperative death rate for Dr. Hawkins last month?

    a. 3.13%

    b. 30.13%

    c. 0.313%

    d. 32%

Use this information to answer questions 288 through 290.
Your physician clinic's CFO has determined that it costs the clinic $3.50 per telephone call for the receptionist to schedule an appointment with a physician in the clinic, compared with $1.50 per online request to schedule an appointment.

288. During one day at the clinic, what would the per appointment cost be if all 250 patient appointments were scheduled by telephone?

    a. $375.00

    b. $525.00

    c. $875.00

    d. $1,325.00

289. During one day at the clinic, what would the per appointment cost be if all 250 patient appointments were scheduled per online request?

    a. $250.00

    b. $375.00

    c. $500.00

    d. $875.00

290. During one day at the clinic, what would the per-appointment cost savings be if 250 patient appointments were arranged by online request rather than by telephone?

    a. $250.00

    b. $375.00

    c. $500.00

    d. $875.00

291. As the COVID-19 pandemic winds down, your CEO wants to know what the hospital can do to prepare for the next epidemic, pandemic, or other natural disaster. She wants information about possible hospital-run testing facilities, hospital pharmacy stockpiling, and extensive PPE training for hospital nursing and ancillary staff. What type of data analytics is being performed in this scenario?

    a. Descriptive analytics

    b. Diagnostic analytics

    c. Predictive analytics

    d. Prescriptive analytics

Use the data in the following table for questions 292 through 294.

Community Hospital Health Information Services Unapproved Abbreviations List November 20XX			
Physician Number	# of Discharges	# of Unapproved Abbreviations	Rate of Unapproved Abbreviations
102	298	34	11.4%
237	247	21	8.5%
391	110	26	23.6%
518	144	22	15.3%
637	206	4	1.9%
802	82	21	25.6%
900	100	12	12.0%
Total	1187	140	

292. After analyzing the data presented in the table, which physician has the highest rate of unapproved abbreviations?

    a. 802

    b. 391

    c. 900

    d. 102

293. After analyzing the data presented in the table, which physician has the highest number of unapproved abbreviations?

    a. 802

    b. 391

    c. 900

    d. 102

294. Using the data presented in the table, calculate the total rate of unapproved abbreviations.

    a. 0.118%

    b. 1.18%

    c. 11.8%

    d. 118%

295. Community Physician's Clinic is a large clinic with 85 physicians. They treat about 9,000 patients each week. Coding professionals are expected to code 100 clinical records each day. How many FTEs are needed to code these records? (Assume a five-day workweek and 7.5 hours as a productive day.)

    a. 7.5 FTEs

    b. 12 FTEs

    c. 17 FTEs

    d. 18 FTEs

296. Two standard deviations from the mean in a normal distribution equals what percent of the area?

    a. 68.26 percent

    b. 95.45 percent

    c. 99.74 percent

    d. 100 percent

297. As you continue research on the COVID-19 pandemic impact on Lakeside Hospital, you discover there is a higher mortality rate in COVID-19 patients due to cerebrovascular accidents. The autopsies show all of these patients suffered from many microinfarcts. What type of data analytics is being performed in this scenario?

    a. Descriptive analytics

    b. Diagnostic analytics

    c. Predictive analytics

    d. Prescriptive analytics

298. An HIM professional is creating a data presentation. The data in the presentation is from the Center for Medicare and Medicaid Services website and illustrates the condition of pneumonia and readmission rates for all hospitals in a specific state. Which of the following is the best choice to graphically display data with this type of focus?

    a. Pareto chart

    b. Pie chart

    c. Line graph

    d. Table

Domain 4 *Revenue Cycle Management*

299. What is the term that means evaluating the appropriateness of the setting for the healthcare service and the level of service?

    a. Coordination of service benefits

    b. Community rating

    c. Outcomes assessment

    d. Utilization review

300. Which of the following actions would be best to determine whether present on admission (POA) indicators for the conditions selected by CMS are having a negative impact on the hospital's Medicare reimbursement?

    a. Identify all records for a period having these indicators for these conditions and determine whether these conditions are the only secondary diagnoses present on the claim that will lead to higher payment.

    b. Identify all records for a period that have these indicators for these conditions.

    c. Identify all records for a period that have these indicators for these conditions and determine whether or not additional documentation can be submitted to Medicare to increase reimbursement.

    d. Take a random sample of records for a period of records having these indicators for these conditions and extrapolate the negative impact on Medicare reimbursement.

301. A patient is admitted to the hospital with acute lower abdominal pain. The principal diagnosis is acute appendicitis. The patient also has a diagnosis of diabetes. The patient undergoes an appendectomy and subsequently develops two wound infections. Which of the following could be considered a comorbid condition?

    a. Acute appendicitis

    b. Acute lower abdominal pain

    c. Diabetes

    d. Wound infection

302. A coding audit shows that an inpatient coding professional is using multiple codes that describe the individual components of a procedure rather than using a single code that describes all the steps of the procedure performed. Which of the following should be done in this case?

    a. Counsel the coding professional and stop the practice immediately.

    b. Report the practice to the OIG.

    c. Require all coding professionals to implement this practice.

    d. Put the coding professional on unpaid leave of absence.

303. NCCI edits prevent improper payments in which of the following cases?

    a. Medical necessity has not been justified by a diagnosis.

    b. The account is potentially upcoded.

    c. The claim contains any of a variety of errors.

    d. Incorrect code combinations are on the claim.

304. Medicare inpatient reimbursement levels are based on:

 a. CPT codes reported during the encounter

 b. MS-DRG calculated for the encounter

 c. Charges accumulated during the episode of care

 d. Usual and customary charges reported during the encounter

305. Dr. Green discharged 30 patients from Medicine Service during the month of August. The given table presents the number of patients discharged by MS-DRG. Calculate the CMI for Dr. Green.

MS-DRG	MS-DRG Title	Rel. Wt.	No. of Pts.	Total Wt. ANSWERS:
179	Respiratory infections and inflammations w/o CC/MCC	0.8727	5	4.3635
187	Pleural effusion w/ CC	1.0329	2	2.0658
189	Pulmonary edema and respiratory failure	1.2261	3	3.6783
194	Simple pneumonia and pleurisy w/ CC	0.8639	1	0.8639
208	Respiratory system diagnosis w/ ventilator support <=96 hours	2.5448	1	2.5448
280	Acute myocardial infarction, discharged alive w/ MCC	1.6069	3	4.8207
299	Peripheral vascular disorders w/ MCC	1.5326	2	3.0652
313	Chest pain	0.7214	4	2.8856
377	G.I. hemorrhage w/ MCC	1.8012	1	1.8012
391	Esophagitis, gastroent. and misc. digest. disorders w/ MCC	1.2492	1	1.2492
547	Connective tissue disorders w/o CC/MCC	0.8336	1	0.8336
552	Medical back problems w/o MCC	0.9434	1	0.9434
684	Renal failure w/o CC/MCC	0.6079	1	0.6079
812	Red blood cell disorders w/o MCC	0.8803	2	1.7606
872	Septicemia w/o MV 96+ hours w/o MCC	1.0263	1	1.0263
918	Poisoning and toxic effects of drugs w/o MCC	0.7916	1	0.7916
Total			30	33.3016

Source: Adapted from McNeill 2020.

 a. 33.3016

 b. 30

 c. 1.110

 d. 2.220

306. A physician query may not be appropriate in which of the following instances?

    a. Diagnosis of viral pneumonia noted in the progress notes and sputum cultures showing *Haemophilus influenzae*

    b. Discharge summary indicates chronic renal failure but the progress notes document acute renal failure throughout the stay

    c. Acute respiratory failure in a patient whose lab report findings appear not to support this diagnosis

    d. Diagnosis of chest pain and abnormal cardiac enzymes indicative of an AMI

307. A 54-year-old patient is seen with a high fever, chest pain, and a cough. Gram stain of the sputum showed staph. The physician documented staphylococcal pneumonia. What code(s) would be assigned for this patient?

B95.7 Other staphylococcus as the cause diseases classified elsewhere

J15.20 Pneumonia due to staphylococcus, unspecified

J18.9 Pneumonia, unspecified organism

R05 Cough

R07.9 Chest pain, unspecified

R50.9 Fever, unspecified

    a. R50.9, R05, R07.9

    b. R50.9, R05, R07.9, J15.20

    c. J15.20

    d. J18.9, B95.7

308. If a patient has an excision of a malignant lesion of the skin, the CPT code is determined by the body area from which the excision occurs and which of the following?

    a. Length of the lesion as described in the pathology report

    b. Dimension of the specimen submitted as described in the pathology report

    c. Width times the length of the lesion as described in the operative report

    d. Diameter of the lesion as well as the margins excised as described in the operative report

309. The present on admission indicator is a requirement for:

    a. Inpatient Medicare claims submitted by hospitals

    b. Inpatient Medicare and Medicaid claims submitted by hospitals

    c. Medicare claims submitted by all entities

    d. Inpatient skilled nursing facility Medicare claims

310. The patient was admitted with nausea, vomiting, and abdominal pain. The physician documents the following on the discharge summary: acute cholecystitis, nausea, vomiting, and abdominal pain. Which of the following would be the correct coding and sequencing for this case?

    a. Acute cholecystitis, nausea, vomiting, abdominal pain

    b. Abdominal pain, vomiting, nausea, acute cholecystitis

    c. Nausea, vomiting, abdominal pain

    d. Acute cholecystitis

311. A patient was admitted for abdominal pain with diarrhea and was diagnosed with infectious gastroenteritis. The patient also had angina and chronic obstructive pulmonary disease. Which of the following would be the correct coding and sequencing for this case?

    a. Abdominal pain; infectious gastroenteritis; chronic obstructive pulmonary disease; angina

    b. Infectious gastroenteritis; chronic obstructive pulmonary disease; angina

    c. Gastroenteritis; abdominal pain; angina

    d. Gastroenteritis; abdominal pain; diarrhea; chronic obstructive pulmonary disease; angina

312. An 80-year-old female is admitted with fever, lethargy, hypotension, tachycardia, oliguria, and elevated WBC. The patient has more than 100,000 organisms of *Escherichia coli* per cc of urine. The attending physician documents "urosepsis." How should this case be coded?

    a. Code sepsis as the principal diagnosis with urinary tract infection due to *E. coli* as secondary diagnosis.

    b. Code urinary tract infection with sepsis as the principal diagnosis.

    c. Query the physician to ask if the patient has septicemia because of the symptomatology.

    d. Query the physician to ask if the patient had septic shock so that this may be used as the principal diagnosis.

313. The practice of using a code that results in a higher payment to the provider than the code that actually reflects the service or item provided is known as:

    a. Unbundling

    b. Billing for services not provided

    c. Medically unnecessary services

    d. Upcoding

314. A 65-year-old patient with a history of lung cancer is admitted to a healthcare facility with ataxia and syncope and a fractured arm as a result of falling. The patient undergoes a closed reduction of the fracture in the emergency department as well as a complete workup for metastatic carcinoma of the brain. The patient is found to have metastatic carcinoma of the lung to the brain and undergoes radiation therapy to the brain. Which of the following would be the principal diagnosis in this case?

    a. Ataxia

    b. Fractured arm

    c. Metastatic carcinoma of the brain

    d. Carcinoma of the lung

315. According to CPT, a repair of a laceration that includes retention sutures would be considered what type of closure?

    a. Complex

    b. Intermediate

    c. Not specified

    d. Simple

316. A patient is admitted with a history of prostate cancer and with mental confusion. The patient completed radiation therapy for prostate carcinoma three years ago and is status post a radical resection of the prostate. CT scan of the brain during the current admission reveals metastasis. Which of the following is the correct coding and sequencing for the current hospital stay?

a. Metastatic carcinoma of the brain; carcinoma of the prostate; mental confusion

b. Mental confusion; history of carcinoma of the prostate; admission for chemotherapy

c. Metastatic carcinoma of the brain; history of carcinoma of the prostate

d. Carcinoma of the prostate; metastatic carcinoma to the brain

317. A patient is admitted with abdominal pain. The physician states that the discharge diagnosis is pancreatitis and noncalculus cholecystitis. Both diagnoses are equally treated. The correct coding and sequencing for this case would be:

a. Either the pancreatitis or noncalculus cholecystitis sequenced as principal diagnosis

b. Pancreatitis; noncalculus cholecystitis; abdominal pain

c. Noncalculus cholecystitis; pancreatitis; abdominal pain

d. Abdominal pain; pancreatitis; noncalculus cholecystitis

318. When coding a benign neoplasm of skin of the vermilion border of the lip, which of the following codes should be used?

> **D10 Benign neoplasm of mouth and pharynx**
> **D10.0 Benign neoplasm of lip**
> Benign neoplasm of lip (frenulum) (inner aspect) (mucosa) (vermilion border)
> *Excludes1:* benign neoplasm of skin of lip (D22.0, D23.0)
> **D10.1 Benign neoplasm of tongue**
> Benign neoplasm of lingual tonsil
> **D10.2 Benign neoplasm of floor of mouth**
> **D23 Other benign neoplasms of skin**
> *Includes:* benign neoplasm of hair follicles
> benign neoplasm of sebaceous glands
> benign neoplasm of sweat glands
> *Excludes1:* benign lipomatous neoplasm of skin (D17.0–D17.3)
> *Excludes2:* melanocytic nevi (D22.-)
> **D23.0 Other benign neoplasm of skin of lip**
> *Excludes1:* benign neoplasm of vermilion border of lip (D10.0)
> **D23.1 Other benign neoplasm of skin of eyelid, including canthus**
> **D23.10 Other benign neoplasm of skin of unspecified eyelid, including canthus**
> **D23.11 Other benign neoplasm of skin of right eyelid, including canthus**
> D23.111 Other benign neoplasm of skin of right upper eyelid, including canthus
> D23.112 Other benign neoplasm of skin of right lower eyelid, including canthus
> **D23.12 Other benign neoplasm of skin of left eyelid, including canthus**
> D23.121 Other benign neoplasm of skin of left upper eyelid, including canthus
> D23.122 Other benign neoplasm of skin of left lower eyelid, including canthus
> **D23.2 Other benign neoplasm of skin of ear and external auricular canal**
> **D23.20 Other benign neoplasm of skin of unspecified ear and external auzcular canal**
> **D23.21 Other benign neoplasm of skin of right ear and external auricular canal**
> **D23.22 Other benign neoplasm of skin of left ear and external auricular canal**

a. D23

b. D10.0

c. D23.0

d. D17.0

319. A seven-year-old patient was admitted to the emergency department for treatment of shortness of breath. The patient is given epinephrine and nebulizer treatments. The shortness of breath and wheezing are unabated following treatment. What diagnosis should be suspected?

    a. Acute bronchitis

    b. Acute bronchitis with chronic obstructive pulmonary disease

    c. Asthma with status asthmaticus

    d. Chronic obstructive asthma

320. The ICD-10-CM utilizes a placeholder character at certain codes to allow for future expansion of the classification system. What letter is used to represent this placeholder character?

    a. A

    b. G

    c. U

    d. X

321. A physician orders a chest x-ray for an office patient who presents with fever, productive cough, and shortness of breath. The physician indicates in the progress notes: "Rule out pneumonia." What should the coding professional report for the visit when the results have not yet been received?

    a. Pneumonia

    b. Fever, cough, shortness of breath

    c. Cough, shortness of breath

    d. Pneumonia, cough, shortness of breath, fever

322. A patient is admitted with spotting. She had been treated two weeks previously for a miscarriage with sepsis. The sepsis had resolved, and she is afebrile at this time. She is treated with an aspiration dilation and curettage. Products of conception are found. Which of the following should be the principal diagnosis?

    a. Miscarriage

    b. Complications of spontaneous abortion with sepsis

    c. Sepsis

    d. Spontaneous abortion with sepsis

323. The capture of secondary diagnoses that increase the incidence of CCs and MCCs at final coding may have an impact on:

    a. Case-mix index

    b. Query rate

    c. Principal diagnosis

    d. Record review rate

324. A 65-year-old woman was admitted to the hospital. She was diagnosed with sepsis secondary to methicillin-susceptible *Staphylococcus aureus* and abdominal pain secondary to diverticulitis of the colon. What is the correct code assignment?

A41.01	Sepsis due to Methicillin susceptible *Staphylococcus aureus*
A41.1	Sepsis due to other specified *Staphylococcus*
A41.2	Sepsis due to unspecified *Staphylococcus*
B95.61	Methicillin susceptible *Staphylococcus aureus* infection as the cause of diseases classified elsewhere
K57.32	Diverticulitis of large intestine without perforation or abscess without bleeding
R10.9	Unspecified abdominal pain

   a. A41.1, K57.32, R10.9

   b. A41.01, K57.32

   c. A41.1, K57.32, B95.61

   d. A41.2, K57.32

325. Use the information provided to determine how much of the APC payment the facility would receive for the status T procedure.

Billing Number	Status Indicator	CPT/HCPCS	APC
998323	V	99285–25	0612
998323	T	25500	0044
998323	X	72050	0261
998323	S	72128	0283
998323	S	70450	0283

   a. 0%

   b. 50%

   c. 75%

   d. 100%

326. Patient was admitted to the hospital and diagnosed with Type 1 diabetic gangrene. What is the correct code assignment?

E10.52	Type 1 diabetes mellitus with diabetic peripheral angiopathy with gangrene
E10.9	Type 1 diabetes mellitus without complication
E11.52	Type 2 diabetes mellitus with diabetic peripheral angiopathy with gangrene
I96	Gangrene, not elsewhere classified

   a. E10.52

   b. E10.9, I96

   c. E10.52, E10.9, I96

   d. E11.52

327. When coding a hydrocystoma of the right upper eyelid, which of the following codes should be used?

> **D10**   **Benign neoplasm of mouth and pharynx**
> **D10.0**   **Benign neoplasm of lip**
>   Benign neoplasm of lip (frenulum) (inner aspect) (mucosa) (vermilion border)
>   *Excludes1:* *benign neoplasm of skin of lip (D22.0, D23.0)*
> **D10.1**   **Benign neoplasm of tongue**
>   Benign neoplasm of lingual tonsil
> **D10.2**   **Benign neoplasm of floor of mouth**
> **D23**   **Other benign neoplasms of skin**
> **Includes:** benign neoplasm of hair follicles
>   benign neoplasm of sebaceous glands
>   benign neoplasm of sweat glands
> *Excludes1:* *benign lipomatous neoplasm of skin (D17.0–D17.3)*
> *Excludes2:* *melanocytic nevi (D22.-)*
> **D23.0**   **Other benign neoplasm of skin of lip**
>   *Excludes1:* *benign neoplasm of vermilion border of lip (D10.0)*
> **D23.1**   **Other benign neoplasm of skin of eyelid, including canthus**
>   **D23.10**   **Other benign neoplasm of skin of unspecified eyelid, including canthus**
>   **D23.11**   **Other benign neoplasm of skin of right eyelid, including canthus**
>   D23.111   Other benign neoplasm of skin of right upper eyelid, including canthus
>   D23.112   Other benign neoplasm of skin of right lower eyelid, including canthus
>   **D23.12**   **Other benign neoplasm of skin of left eyelid, including canthus**
>   D23.121   Other benign neoplasm of skin of left upper eyelid, including canthus
>   D23.122   Other benign neoplasm of skin of left lower eyelid, including canthus
> **D23.2**   **Other benign neoplasm of skin of ear and external auricular canal**
>   **D23.20**   **Other benign neoplasm of skin of unspecified ear and external auzcular canal**
>   **D23.21**   **Other benign neoplasm of skin of right ear and external auricular canal**
>   **D23.22**   **Other benign neoplasm of skin of left ear and external auricular canal**

a. D23

b. D17.0

c. D23.121

d. D23.111

328. Identify the two-digit modifier that may be reported to indicate a physician performed the postoperative management of a patient but another physician performed the surgical procedure.

a. -22, Increased procedural services

b. -54, Surgical care only

c. -32, Mandated service

d. -55, Postoperative management only

329. Assign the correct CPT code for the following procedure: Revision of the pacemaker skin pocket.

a. 33223, Relocation of skin pocket for implantable defibrillator

b. 33210, Insertion or replacement of temporary transvenous single chamber cardiac electrode or pacemaker catheter (separate procedure)

c. 33212, Insertion of pacemaker pulse generator only; with existing single lead

d. 33222, Relocation of skin pocket for pacemaker

330. In the inpatient prospective payment system, the calculation of the DRG begins with the:

    a. Principal diagnosis

    b. Primary diagnosis

    c. Secondary diagnosis

    d. Surgical procedure

331. Assign the correct CPT code for the following: A 63-year-old female had a temporal artery biopsy completed in the outpatient surgical center.

    a. 32408, Core needle biopsy, lung or mediastinum, percutaneous, including imaging guidance, when performed

    b. 37609, Ligation or biopsy, temporal artery

    c. 20206, Biopsy, muscle, percutaneous needle

    d. 31629, Bronchoscopy, rigid or flexible, including fluoroscopic guidance, when performed; with transbronchial needle aspiration biopsy(s), trachea, main stem and/or lobar bronchus(i)

332. In ICD-10-PCS, the root operation defined as taking or letting out fluids and/or gases from a body part is:

    a. Control

    b. Drainage

    c. Excision

    d. Release

333. When reporting an encounter for a patient who is HIV positive but has never had any symptoms, the following code is assigned:

    a. B20, Human immunodeficiency virus [HIV] disease

    b. Z21, Asymptomatic human immunodeficiency virus [HIV] infection status

    c. R75, Inconclusive laboratory evidence of human immunodeficiency virus [HIV]

    d. Z20.6, Contact with and (suspected) exposure to human immunodeficiency virus [HIV]

334. What is the name of the process to determine whether medical care provided to a specific patient is necessary according to pre-established objective screening criteria at time frames specified?

    a. Case management

    b. Continuum of care

    c. Quality improvement

    d. Utilization review

335. What type of value-based purchasing program is the Hospital-Acquired Conditions Reduction Program?

    a. Quality consumer assessment

    b. Pay for reporting

    c. Quality incentive program

    d. Paying for value

336. Under outpatient prospective payment system, Medicare decides how much a hospital or a community mental health center will be reimbursed for each service rendered. Depending on the service, the patient pays either a coinsurance amount (20 percent) or a fixed copayment amount, whichever is less. Mr. Smith had a minor procedure performed in the hospital outpatient department at a charge of $85. In addition, Mr. Smith has paid his deductible for the year. The fixed copayment amount for this type of procedure, adjusted for wages in the geographic area, is $15. What would Mr. Smith need to pay in this case?

    a. $15

    b. $17

    c. $68

    d. $85

337. Which of the following is the condition established after study to be the reason for hospitalization?

    a. Principal procedure

    b. Complication

    c. Comorbidity

    d. Principal diagnosis

338. MS-DRGs may be split into a maximum of _____ payment tiers based on severity as determined by the presence of a major complication or comorbidity, a CC, or no CC.

    a. Two

    b. Three

    c. Four

    d. Five

339. The purpose of the present on admission indicator is to:

    a. Differentiate between conditions present on admission and conditions that develop during an inpatient admission

    b. Track principal diagnoses

    c. Distinguish between principal and primary diagnoses

    d. Determine principal diagnosis

340. What is the procedure code for a patient who had ventilator management for more than 96 hours in ICD-10-PCS?

Section	5	Extracorporeal or Systemic Assistance and Performance		
Body System	A	Physiological systems		
Operation	1	Performance: Completely taking over a physiological function by extracorporeal means		

Body System	Duration	Function	Qualifier
2 Cardiac	**0** Single	**1** Output	**2** Manual
2 Cardiac	**1** Intermittent	**3** Pacing	**Z** No Qualifier
2 Cardiac	**2** Continuous	**1** Output	**Z** No Qualifier
2 Cardiac	**2** Continuous	**3** Pacing	**Z** No Qualifier
5 Circulatory	**2** Continuous	**2** Oxygenation	**F** Membrane, Central **G** Membrane, Peripheral Veno-aterial **H** Membrane, Peripheral Veno-venous
9 Respiratory	**0** Single	**5** Ventilation	**4** Nonmechanical
9 Respiratory	**3** Less than 24 Consecutive Hours **4** 24–96 Consecutive Hours **5** Greater than 96 Consecutive Hours	**5** Ventilation	**Z** No Qualifier
C Biliary	**0** Single **6** Multiple	**0** Filtration	**Z** No Qualifier
D Urinary	**7** Intermittent, Less than 6 Hours Per Day **8** Prolonged Intermittent, 6–18 Hours Per Day **9** Continuous, Greater than 18 Hours Per Day	**0** Filtration	**Z** No Qualifier

a. 5A1955Z

b. 5A1945Z

c. 5A09557

d. 5A09458

341. The coding supervisor has compiled a report on the number of coding errors made each day by the coding staff. The report data show that Tim makes an average of six errors per day, Jane makes an average of five errors per day, and Bob and Susan each make an average of two errors per day. Given this information, what immediate action should the coding supervisor take?

a. Counsel Tim and Jane because they have the highest error rates.

b. Encourage Tim and Jane to get additional training.

c. Provide Bob and Susan with incentive pay for a low coding error rate.

d. Take no action because not enough information is given to make a judgment.

342. The National Correct Coding Initiative (NCCI) was developed to control improper coding leading to inappropriate payment for:

a. Part A Medicare claims

b. Part B Medicare claims

c. Medicaid claims

d. Medicare and Medicaid claims

343. A quality data review based on specific problem areas that comes after an initial baseline review has been completed in a hospital is called a:

    a. Compliance initiative

    b. Concurrent review

    c. Focused review

    d. Internal audit

344. Unbundling refers to:

    a. Use of a comprehensive code to appropriately maximize reimbursement

    b. Use of multiple procedure codes when a comprehensive code is available

    c. Combined billing for pre- and postsurgery physician services

    d. Using the incorrect DRG code

345. A patient who has been diagnosed with hypertension visits her physician on a monthly basis. The nurse conducted the blood pressure check under the physician's supervision. Code the office visit.

    a. 99211, Office or other outpatient visit of the evaluation and management of an established patient that may not require the presence of a physician or other qualified healthcare professional.

    b. 99202, Office or other outpatient visit for the evaluation and management of a new patient, which requires a medically appropriate history and/or examination and straightforward medical decision.

    c. 99203, Office or other outpatient visit for the evaluation and management of a new patient, which requires a medically appropriate history and/or examination and low level of medical decision making.

    d. 99212, Office or other outpatient visit for the evaluation and management of an established patient, which requires a medically appropriate history and/or examination and straightforward medical decision.

346. In the healthcare industry, what is the term for the written report that insurers use to notify insureds about the extent of payments made on a claim?

    a. Certificate of Insurance

    b. Coordination of Benefits

    c. Explanation of Benefits

    d. Summary of Benefits and Coverage

347. You are the coding supervisor, and you are doing an audit of outpatient coding. Robert Thompson was seen in the outpatient department with a chronic cough and the record states, "rule out lung cancer." What should have been coded as the patient's diagnosis?

    a. Chronic cough

    b. Observation and evaluation without need for further medical care

    c. Diagnosis of unknown etiology

    d. Lung cancer

348. The patient was admitted to the outpatient department and had a bronchoscopy with bronchial brushings performed. What is the appropriate code assignment?

> | 31622 | Bronchoscopy, rigid or flexible, including fluoroscopic guidance, when performed, diagnostic, with cell washing when performed (separate procedure) |
> |-------|---|
> | 31623 | Bronchoscopy, rigid or flexible, including fluoroscopic guidance, when performed; with brushing or protected brushings |
> | 31625 | Bronchoscopy, rigid or flexible, including fluoroscopic guidance, when performed; with bronchial or endobronchial biopsy(s), single or multiple sites |
> | 31640 | Bronchoscopy, rigid or flexible, including fluoroscopic guidance, when performed; with excision of tumor |

    a. 31622, 31640

    b. 31622, 31623

    c. 31623

    d. 31625

349. The function of the NCCI editor is to:

    a. Report poor performing physicians

    b. Identify procedures and services that cannot be billed together on the same day of service for a patient

    c. Identify poor performing coding professionals

    d. Identify problems in the national coding system

350. A select group of reasonably preventable conditions for which hospitals should not receive additional payment when one of the conditions was not present on admission is called a:

    a. Charge code

    b. Hospital-acquired condition

    c. Principal diagnosis

    d. Value-based purchasing list

351. When multiple burns are present, the first sequenced diagnosis is the:

    a. Burn that is treated surgically

    b. Burn that is closest to the head

    c. Highest-degree burn

    d. Burn that is treated first

352. The results of a recent coding audit show that two of the inpatient coding professionals are missing the correct principal diagnosis selection that affects MS-DRG payment for the hospital. As the coding manager, you are tasked to provide coding education to the coding professionals to correct this problem. What should be included in this training?

    a. How to use the CPT index

    b. Definitions of root operations

    c. How to calculate the case mix

    d. Definitions of principal diagnosis

353. A patient known to have AIDS is admitted to the hospital for treatment of *Pneumocystis carinii* pneumonia. Assign the principal diagnosis for this patient.

    a. B20, Human immunodeficiency virus [HIV] disease

    b. J18.9, Pneumonia, unspecified organism

    c. B59, Pneumocystosis

    d. Z21, Asymptomatic human immunodeficiency virus [HIV] infection status

354. A patient is seen as an outpatient to receive chemotherapy for distal esophageal carcinoma. What is the appropriate first-listed diagnosis?

    a. Z48.3, Aftercare following surgery for neoplasm

    b. Z51.11, Encounter for antineoplastic chemotherapy

    c. C15.5, Malignant neoplasm of lower third of esophagus

    d. C15.3, Malignant neoplasm of upper third of esophagus

355. The discharged, not final billed report (also known as "discharged, no final bill" or "accounts not selected for billing") includes what types of accounts?

    a. Accounts that have been discharged and have not been billed for a variety of reasons

    b. Only discharged inpatient accounts awaiting generation of the bill

    c. Only uncoded patient records

    d. Accounts that are within the system hold days and not eligible to be billed

356. NCCI edit files contain code pairs, called mutually exclusive edits, that prevent payment for:

    a. Services that cannot reasonably be billed together

    b. Services that are components of a more comprehensive procedure

    c. Unnecessary procedures

    d. Comprehensive procedures

357. What is the benefit to comparing the coding assigned by coding professionals to the coding appearing on the claim?

    a. May find that more codes are required to support the claim

    b. May find that the charge description master soft coding is inaccurate

    c. Serves as a way for HIM to take over the management of patient financial services

    d. Could find claim generation issues that cannot be found other ways

358. A clinical documentation improvement (CDI) program facilitates accurate coding and helps coding professionals avoid:

    a. NCCI edits

    b. Upcoding

    c. Coding without a completed face sheet

    d. Assumption coding

359. When the physician does not specify the method used to remove a lesion during an endoscopy, what is the appropriate procedure?

    a. Assign the removal by snare technique code.

    b. Assign the removal by hot biopsy forceps code.

    c. Assign the ablation code.

    d. Query the physician as to the method used.

360. A 27-year-old female has a vaginal delivery with single liveborn female at 40-weeks gestation with episiotomy and repair. What diagnosis and procedure codes would be assigned for this patient?

O70.0	First degree perineal laceration during delivery
O70.9	Perineal laceration during delivery, unspecified
O80	Encounter for full-term uncomplicated delivery
Z37.0	Single live birth
Z3A.40	40 weeks of gestation of pregnancy

Section	Body System	Root Operation	Body Part	Approach	Device	Qualifier
Medical and Surgical	Anatomical Regions, General	Division	Perineum, Female	External	No Device	No Qualifier
0	W	8	N	X	Z	Z

Section	Body System	Root Operation	Body Part	Approach	Device	Qualifier
Medical and Surgical	Anatomical Regions, General	Repair	Perineum, Female	External	No Device	No Qualifier
0	W	Q	N	X	Z	Z

    a. O70.0, Z37.0, Z3A.40, 0WQNXZZ

    b. O80, Z37.0, Z3A.40, 0W8NXZZ, 0WQNXZZ

    c. O80, Z37.0, Z3A.40, 0W8NXZZ

    d. O70.9. Z37.0, 0WQNXZZ

361. The hospital-acquired conditions provision of the Medicare PPS is an example of which type of value-based purchasing system?

    a. Paying for value

    b. Penalty-based

    c. Reward-based

    d. Penalty for value

362. Which of the following would be classified in ICD-10-CM with an external cause code?

    a. Echocardiogram

    b. Fall from curb

    c. Adenocarcinoma

    d. Admission for plastic surgery

363. A patient is scheduled for an outpatient colonoscopy, but due to a sudden drop in blood pressure, the procedure is canceled just as the scope is introduced into the rectum. Because of moderately severe mental retardation, the patient is given general anesthetic prior to the procedure. How should this procedure be coded?

    a. Assign the code for colonoscopy with modifier 74, Discontinued outpatient procedure after anesthesia administration.

    b. Assign the code for a colonoscopy with modifier 52, Reduced services.

    c. Assign no code because no procedure was performed.

    d. Assign an anesthesia code only.

364. When documentation in the health record is not clear, the coding professional should:

    a. Submit the question to the coding clinic.

    b. Refer to dictation from other encounters for the patient to get clarification.

    c. Query the physician who originated the progress note or other report in question.

    d. Query a physician who consistently responds to queries in a timely manner.

365. Which of the following procedures or services could *not* be assigned a code with CPT?

    a. Gastroscopy

    b. Anesthesia

    c. Glucose tolerance test

    d. Crutches

366. Which of the following would generally be found in a query to a physician?

    a. Health record number and demographic information

    b. Name and contact number of the individual initiating the query and account number

    c. Date query initiated and date query must be completed

    d. Demographic information and name and contact number of the individual initiating the query

367. In ICD-10-PCS, what is the root operation for a left heart catheterization with sampling and pressure measurement?

    a. Insertion

    b. Introduction

    c. Measurement

    d. Monitoring

368. The pathologist performed a gross and microscopic examination of a kidney biopsy. What is the correct CPT code assignment?

88300	Level I, Surgical pathology, gross examination only
88305	Level IV, Surgical pathology, gross and microscopic examination
88307	Level V, Surgical pathology, gross and microscopic examination

    a. 88300, 88305

    b. 88305

    c. 88307

    d. 88300, 88307

369. When assigning evaluation and management codes for hospital outpatient services, the coding professional should follow:

   a. The hospital's own internal guidelines

   b. AHIMA guidelines

   c. CMS guidelines

   d. AHA guidelines

370. The physician performs an exploratory laparotomy with bilateral salpingo-oophorectomy. What is the correct CPT code assignment for this procedure?

49000	Exploratory laparotomy, exploratory celiotomy with or without biopsy(s) (separate procedure)
58700	Salpingectomy, complete or partial, unilateral or bilateral (separate procedure)
58720	Salpingo-oophorectomy, complete or partial, unilateral or bilateral (separate procedure)
58940	Oophorectomy, partial or total, unilateral or bilateral
-50	Bilateral procedure

   a. 49000, 58940, 58700

   b. 58940, 58720-50

   c. 49000, 58720

   d. 58720

371. Code the following scenario: Patient with flank pain was admitted and found to have a calculus of the left kidney. Ureteroscopy with placement of bilateral ureteral stents was performed.

N20.0	Calculus of kidney
N20.2	Calculus of kidney with calculus of ureter
N20.9	Urinary calculus, unspecified
R10.9	Unspecified abdominal pain

Section	Body System	Root Operation	Body Part	Approach	Device	Qualifier
Medical and Surgical	Urinary System	Dilation	Ureters, Bilateral	Via Natural or Artificial Opening Endoscopic	Intraluminal Device	No Qualifier
0	T	7	8	8	D	Z

Section	Body System	Root Operation	Body Part	Approach	Device	Qualifier
Medical and Surgical	Urinary System	Insertion	Ureter	Via Natural or Artificial Opening Endoscopic	Infusion Device	No Qualifier
0	T	H	9	8	3	Z

   a. N20.0, 0T788DZ, 0TH983Z

   b. N20.2, N20.9, 0T788DZ

   c. N20.0, 0TH983Z

   d. N20.0, 0T788DZ

372. The main purpose of National Correct Coding Initiative edits is to prohibit:

    a. ICD-10-CM procedure code errors

    b. DRG assignment errors

    c. Unbundling of procedures

    d. Incorrect POA assignment

373. Patient admitted with chronic cystitis. A cystoscopy and biopsy of the bladder were performed. What diagnosis and procedure codes would be assigned for this patient?

N30.10	Interstitial cystitis (chronic) without hematuria
N30.20	Other chronic cystitis without hematuria
N30.30	Trigonitis without hematuria
N39.0	Urinary tract infection, site not specified

Section	Body System	Root Operation	Body Part	Approach	Device	Qualifier
Medical and Surgical	Urinary System	Inspection	Bladder	Via Natural or Artificial Opening Endoscopic	No Device	No Qualifier
0	T	J	B	8	Z	Z

Section	Body System	Root Operation	Body Part	Approach	Device	Qualifier
Medical and Surgical	Urinary System	Excision	Bladder	Via Natural or Artificial Opening Endoscopic	No Device	Diagnostic
0	T	B	B	8	Z	X

    a. N30.30, 0TBB8ZX

    b. N30.20, 0TBB8ZX, 0TJB8ZZ

    c. N30.20, 0TBB8ZX

    d. N39.0, 0TBB8ZX

374. Date of service: 1/3/2022. Last date of treatment: 2/12/2021. The patient is seen in the physician's office for a cough and sore throat. The physician performs a medically appropriate examination, and medical decision-making is straightforward. What is the correct E/M code for this service?

    a. 99213, Office or other outpatient visit for the evaluation and management of an established patient, which requires a medically appropriate history and/or examination and low level of medical decision making

    b. 99212, Office or other outpatient visit for the evaluation and management of an established patient, which requires a medically appropriate history and/or examination and straightforward decision making

    c. 99214, Office or other outpatient visit for the evaluation and management of an established patient, which requires a medically appropriate history and/or examination and moderate level of medical decision making

    d. 99211, Office or other outpatient visit of the evaluation and management of an established patient that may not require the presence of a physician or other healthcare professional

375. What is the correct CPT code assignment for hysteroscopy with lysis of intrauterine adhesions?

58555	Hysteroscopy, diagnostic (separate procedure)
58559	Hysteroscopy, surgical; with lysis of intrauterine adhesions (any method)
58740	Lysis of adhesions (salpingolysis, ovariolysis)

    a. 58555, 58559

    b. 58559

    c. 58559, 58740

    d. 58555, 58559, 58740

376. Assign codes for the following scenario: A female patient is admitted for stress incontinence. A urethral suspension is performed.

N23	Unspecified renal colic
N39.3	Stress incontinence (female) (male)
R32	Unspecified urinary incontinence

Section	Body System	Root Operation	Body Part	Approach	Device	Qualifier
Medical and Surgical	Urinary System	Reposition	Urethra	Open	No Device	No Qualifier
0	T	S	D	0	Z	Z

Section	Body System	Root Operation	Body Part	Approach	Device	Qualifier
Medical and Surgical	Urinary System	Supplement	Urethra	Open	Synthetic Substitute	No Qualifier
0	T	U	D	0	J	Z

    a. N39.3, 0TUD0JZ

    b. N23, 0TSD0ZZ

    c. N39.3, 0TSD0ZZ

    d. R32, 0TUD0JZ

377. Which of the following statements best defines utilization management?

    a. It is the process of determining whether the medical care provided to a patient is necessary.

    b. It is a set of processes used to determine the appropriateness of medical services provided during specific episodes of care.

    c. It is a process that determines whether a planned service or a patient's condition warrants care in an inpatient setting.

    d. It is an ongoing infection surveillance program.

378. All of the following are steps in medical necessity and utilization review, *except*:

    a. Initial clinical review

    b. Peer clinical review

    c. Access consideration

    d. Appeals consideration

379. A patient was admitted to the hospital for treatment of a myocardial infarction (heart attack) and the MS-DRG assigned was 236 Coronary bypass w/o cardiac cath w/o MCC. During the patient's admission, a bypass procedure was performed on day 2; on day 4, the patient was diagnosed with sepsis, which was not present on admission. Sepsis is a major complication. This case was identified as coded incorrectly in a recent audit by the coding manager. What was the error that was made by the coding professional?

    a. The sepsis was not coded, and so an MCC was missed.

    b. The coronary bypass procedure was coded incorrectly.

    c. The claim was coded correctly; no error was made.

    d. The cardiac catheterization procedure was not coded.

380. Which of the following services is most likely to be considered medically necessary?

    a. Caregivers' convenience or relief

    b. Cosmetic improvement

    c. Investigational cancer prevention

    d. Standard of care for health condition

381. In processing a bill under the Medicare outpatient prospective payment system (OPPS) in which a patient had three surgical procedures with the payment status indicator T performed during the same operative session, which of the following would apply?

    a. Bundling of services

    b. Discounting of procedures

    c. Outlier adjustment

    d. Pass-through payment

382. When a service is not considered medically necessary based on the reason for encounter, the patient should be provided with a(n) _____ indicating that Medicare might not pay and that the patient might be responsible for the entire charge.

    a. OIG

    b. ABN

    c. LOS

    d. EOB

383. The period of time between discharge and claim submission, which a facility defines by policy, is called the:

    a. AR days

    b. Bill hold

    c. Cash flow days

    d. Denial period

384. When an obstetric patient enters the hospital for complications of pregnancy during one trimester and remains in the hospital into a subsequent trimester, the final character in ICD-10-CM selected for the antepartum condition should be:

a. For the trimester in which the complication developed

b. For the trimester in which the patient delivered

c. For the trimester in which the patient was discharged

d. For any trimester as long as the same character is used for all complications

385. In order to determine the hospital's expected MS-DRG payment, the hospital's blended rate is multiplied by the MS-DRG's _____ to determine the dollar amount paid.

a. Length of stay

b. Case-mix number

c. Relative weight

d. Major diagnostic category

386. Which of the following is the average relative weight of all cases treated at a given facility or by a given physician?

a. Case-mix index

b. Sampling

c. Hospital-acquired condition

d. Present on admission indicator

387. A patient has been discharged prior to an administrative utilization review being conducted. Which of the following should be performed?

a. Continued stay utilization review

b. Discharge plan

c. Retrospective utilization review

d. Case management

388. The evaluation of coding professionals is recommended at least quarterly for the purpose of measurement and assurance of:

a. Speed

b. Data quality and integrity

c. Accuracy

d. Effective relationships with physicians and facility personnel

389. The quality improvement organizations (QIOs) under contract with CMS conduct audits on high-risk and hospital-specific data from claims data in which of the following?

a. Hospital Payment Monitoring Program

b. Payment Error Prevention Program

c. Program for Evaluation Payment Patterns Electronic Report

d. Compliance Program Guidance for Hospitals

390. Community Hospital has launched a clinical documentation improvement (CDI) initiative. Currently, clinical documentation does not always adequately reflect the severity of illness of the patient or support optimal HIM coding accuracy. Given this situation, which of the following would be the best action to validate that the new program is achieving its goals?

    a. Hire clinical documentation specialists to review records prior to coding.

    b. Ask coding professionals to query physicians more often.

    c. Provide physicians the opportunity to add addenda to their reports to clarify documentation issues.

    d. Conduct a retrospective review of all query opportunities for the year.

391. In a typical acute-care setting, the Explanation of Benefits (EOB), Medicare Summary Notice (MSN), and Remittance Advice (RA) documents (provided by the payer) are monitored in which revenue cycle area?

    a. Preclaims submission

    b. Claims processing

    c. Claims reconciliation and collections

    d. Accounts receivable

392. A facility recently submitted two claims for the same service for a patient's recent encounter for chemotherapy. If the third-party payer pays both of these claims, the facility will receive a higher reimbursement than deserved. This is called:

    a. Appropriate payment

    b. Overpayment

    c. Unbundling

    d. Waste

393. Which of the following would *not* be a focus area of claims auditing for healthcare services provided in the emergency department?

    a. Ensuring claims are not submitted more than once

    b. Ensuring procedures are reported at the appropriate level

    c. Ensuring documentation supports services reported on the claim

    d. Ensuring patients are satisfied with their services

394. The clinical documentation improvement (CDI) program must keep high-quality records of the query process for:

    a. Revenue cycle analysis

    b. Compliance issues

    c. Chart deficiency tracking

    d. Reducing the workload on HIM

395. Detailed query documentation can be used to:

    a. Protect the hospital from lawsuits

    b. Protect the hospital against claims from physicians about leading queries

    c. Show the effects of follow-up training

    d. Protect the auditor from corrective action

396. If a patient notices an unknown item in the explanation of benefits they receive from an insurance company and they do not recognize the service being paid for, the patient should:

a. Contact the insurer and the provider who billed for the services to correct the information.

b. Contact the police.

c. Contact human resources and let them know there has been a mistake.

d. Not do anything.

397. Insurance companies pool premium payments for all the insureds in a group, then use actuarial data to calculate the group's premiums so that which of the following occurs?

a. Premium payments are lowered for insurance plan payers.

b. The pool is large enough to pay losses of the entire group.

c. Accounting for the group's plan is simplified.

d. Insurance companies are guaranteed to never have a loss.

398. When a provider does not accept the amount paid by the healthcare insurance plan and requires the patient to pay the remaining charges of a service, this is called:

a. Accept assignment

b. Bundled payment

c. Balanced billing

d. Capitated payment

399. Midwest Healthcare Insurance has a contract with Memorial Hospital for inpatient surgical admissions. They have agreed to a case rate methodology for these admissions. The case rate for a coronary artery bypass graft surgical admission is $28,500. Memorial Hospital submitted claims for the following admissions.

Admission #	Surgery	LOS	Charges	Cost
123	Coronary artery bypass graft	5	$78,050	$27,317
124	Coronary artery bypass graft	6	$84,400	$29,540
126	Coronary artery bypass graft	5	$79,450	$27,808

What is the total reimbursement Memorial Hospital will receive for each admission?

a. $28,500

b. $84,665

c. $241,900

d. $456,000

400. Which of the following is *not* a reason to query a provider?

a. To clear up ambiguous documentation

b. If conflicting information is found between the documentation of two different providers

c. If the documentation is incomplete

d. To question why a physician would document a condition

401. Dr. Jones is a podiatrist who performs over 100 bunionectomies a year. Western Health Insurance insures several of Dr. Jones' patients. Western Health Insurance reimburses Dr. Jones one amount for the preoperative visit, the surgery, and routine postoperative follow-up visits. Which reimbursement methodology does Western Health Insurance use to reimburse Dr. Jones?

    a. Global payment method

    b. Fee schedule

    c. Case-rate methodology

    d. Prospective payment methodology

402. Using the data displayed here, calculate the March 20XX CC/MCC capture rate for the chronic obstructive pulmonary disease MS-DRG family.

MS-DRG Family Chronic Obstructive Pulmonary Disease Admission Data for March 20XX		
MS-DRG	**MS-DRG Description**	**Admission Volume**
190	Chronic obstructive pulmonary disease with MCC	15
191	Chronic obstructive pulmonary disease with CC	25
192	Chronic obstructive pulmonary disease without CC/MCC	30

    a. 21.4%

    b. 35.7%

    c. 42.8%

    d. 57.1%

Use the following scenario for questions 403 and 404.

Dr. Gilbert sees a 14-year-old male with adolescent idiopathic thoracic scoliosis. Surgery for spinal fusion was canceled after the patient was diagnosed with mononucleosis. On today's visit the patient is started on prednisone for severe sore throat and difficulty swallowing. The patient was accompanied by his parents who have health insurance through the mother's employment at the State Department of Treasury.

403. Who is the first party in this healthcare reimbursement scenario?

    a. Patient

    b. Parents

    c. Dr. Gilbert

    d. Insurance company

404. Who is the second party in this healthcare reimbursement scenario?

    a. Patient

    b. Parents

    c. Dr. Gilbert

    d. Society

405. Which key performance indicator (KPI) measures the effectiveness of coding management?

  a. Case-mix index

  b. Denial rate

  c. Clean claim rate

  d. Discharged, not final billed

406. How many times is a CDI specialist required to examine a patient's medical record documentation prior to the patient being discharged or transferred?

  a. Once, on the last day of the admission

  b. Twice, on the first and last days of the admission

  c. As many times as the admission length of stay

  d. As many times as warranted based on the clinical documentation and circumstances of the admission

407. Kyle is the CDI supervisor at University Hospital. He is reviewing data for the month of March. There were 215 discharges available for review in March. His CDI team was able to review 174. What is the review rate for March?

  a. 1.24%

  b. 44.7%

  c. 80.9%

  d. Cannot determine because the number of CDI professionals is not provided

408. Which of the following would be considered a back-end process of the revenue cycle?

  a. Adjudication

  b. Prior authorization

  c. Charge capture

  d. Diagnosis of coding

409. Which of the following sections in the ICD-10-PCS coding system contains codes for services that are new to ICD-10-PCS or that capture services not routinely captured in ICD-10-PCS that have been presented for public comment at the Coordination and Maintenance Committee Meeting?

  a. Other Procedures

  b. New Technology

  c. New Procedures

  d. Other Technology

410. On a CMS-1500 billing form, linking refers to which of the following?

  a. Attaching modifiers to CPT codes

  b. Substituting a HCPCS code for the appropriate CPT code

  c. Assigning a diagnosis code to a CPT code on a claim

  d. Pairing professional charges to technical charges on a claim

411. A code used to describe what a patient was doing at the time of injury or other health condition occurred is called:

    a. External cause status code

    b. Place of occurrence code

    c. External cause code

    d. Activity code

412. What is the function of a clearinghouse?

    a. It ensures that computer viruses are removed from billing software.

    b. It manages the process of claims appeals for Medicare.

    c. It reprices claims for a physician network.

    d. It transfers electronic claims to individual insurers.

413. Gloria is the CDI supervisor at Memorial Hospital. She is reviewing data for the month of October. The CDI team sent 35 requests to physicians for clarification on severity. Twenty-one of these clarifications increased or impacted the MS-DRG assignment. What is the physician clarification impact rate for October?

    a. 14%

    b. 56%

    c. 60%

    d. 735%

414. Dr. Smith submitted 130 claims for code 36415 during the past year. The claim history file shows:

    36415 $8.25 — 10 claims
    36415 $8.75 — 20 claims
    36415 $9.25 — 100 claims

    What is Dr. Smith's fee profile for 36415, using usual and customary (U/C) rules?

    a. $8.25

    b. $8.75

    c. $9.10

    d. $9.25

415. What do insurance companies receive in return for assuming the insured's exposure to risk or loss?

    a. Bonus

    b. Stipend

    c. Formulary

    d. Premium

416. Dr. Anderson is a gynecologist who performs surgery at City Hospital. She performs approximately 15 surgeries per month. Her office staff generates claims for her surgeries. What coding system should her staff use to code the surgeries on the provider (physician) claim?

   a. CPT

   b. SNOMED CT

   c. ICD-10-PCS

   d. CDT4

Domain 5   *Compliance*

417. Which of the following is *not* part of healthcare fraud?

   a. Damage to another party that reasonably relied on misrepresentation

   b. False representation of fact

   c. Failure to disclose a material fact

   d. Unnecessary costs to a program

418. Corporate compliance programs became common after adoption of which of the following?

   a. False Claims Act

   b. Federal Sentencing Guidelines

   c. Fair Labor Standards Act

   d. Federal Physician Self-Referral Statute

419. A group practice has hired an HIT as its chief compliance officer. The current compliance program includes written standards of conduct and policies, and procedures that address specific areas of potential fraud. It also has audits in place to monitor compliance. Which of the following should the compliance officer also ensure are in place?

   a. A bonus program for coding professionals who code charts with higher paying MS-DRGs

   b. A hotline to receive complaints and adoption of procedures to protect whistleblowers from retaliation

   c. Procedures to adequately identify individuals who make complaints so that appropriate follow-up can be conducted

   d. A corporate compliance committee that reports directly to the CFO

420. Which of the following is not an example of a high-risk billing practice that creates compliance risks for healthcare organizations?

   a. Altered claim forms

   b. Returned overpayments

   c. Duplicate billings

   d. Unbundled procedures

421. Which of the following entities issues compliance program guidance?

    a. AHIMA

    b. CMS

    c. *Federal Register*

    d. HHS Office of Inspector General

422. In developing a coding compliance program, which of the following would *not* be ordinarily included as participants in coding compliance education?

    a. Current coding personnel

    b. Medical staff

    c. Newly hired coding personnel

    d. Nursing staff

423. The Medicare Integrity Program was established to battle fraud and abuse and is charged with which of the following responsibilities?

    a. Audit of expense reports and notifying beneficiaries of their rights

    b. Payment determinations and audit of cost reports

    c. Publishing of new coding guidelines and code changes

    d. Monitoring of physician credentials and payment determinations

424. Insufficient documentation is the highest risk area for physician services. Which of the following is the best approach for the coding supervisor at Family Physicians group to combat this issue?

    a. Ensure medical record documentation is submitted for every single CERT record request.

    b. Work with billing to ensure only valid CPT and HCPCS codes are reported on Medicare claims.

    c. Design and execute a physician documentation assessment.

    d. Perform a root cause analysis of records denied for insufficient documentation and then develop a plan based on the findings.

425. If an HIM department acts in deliberate ignorance or in disregard of official coding guidelines, it may be committing:

    a. Abuse

    b. Fraud

    c. Malpractice

    d. Kickbacks

426. In Medicare, which of the following is *not* one of the most common forms of fraud and abuse?

    a. Billing for services not furnished

    b. Misrepresenting the diagnosis to justify payment

    c. Unbundling or exploding charges

    d. Implementing a clinical documentation improvement program

427. Which of the following should not be included in the policies and procedures section of a coding compliance plan?

   a. Physician query process

   b. Unbundling

   c. Assignment of discharge disposition codes

   d. Utilization review

428. When the Medicare Recovery Audit Contractor has determined that incorrect payment has been made to an organization, which document is sent to the provider notifying them of this determination?

   a. Appeal request

   b. Claims denial

   c. Demand letter

   d. Medicare Summary Notice

429. Which of the following is an example of a common form of healthcare fraud and abuse?

   a. Billing for services not furnished to patients

   b. Clinical documentation improvement

   c. Refiling claims after denials

   d. Use of a claim scrubber prior to submitting bills

430. Every healthcare organization's risk management plan does not have to include which of the following components?

   a. Loss prevention and reduction

   b. Risk identification and analysis

   c. Peer review

   d. Claims management

431. Which of the following should be the first step in any quality improvement process?

   a. Analyze the problem.

   b. Identify the performance measures.

   c. Develop an alternative solution.

   d. Decide on the best solution.

432. An organization accredited by the Joint Commission must review its formulary annually to ensure a medication's continued:

   a. Safety and dose

   b. Efficiency and efficacy

   c. Efficacy and safety

   d. Dose and efficiency

433. From an evidentiary standpoint, incident reports:

    a. Are universally nonadmissible during trial proceedings

    b. May be referenced in the patient's health record

    c. Should not be placed in a patient's health record

    d. Are universally nondiscoverable during litigation

434. A hospital employee destroyed a health record so that its contents—which would be damaging to the employee—could not be used at trial. In legal terms, the employee's action constitutes:

    a. Mutilation

    b. Destruction

    c. Spoliation

    d. Spoilage

435. Per the HITECH breach notification requirements, what is the threshold for the immediate notification of each individual?

    a. 1,000 individuals affected

    b. 500 individuals affected

    c. 250 individuals affected

    d. Any number of individuals affected requires individual notification.

436. Which of the following is *not* a measure used to track and assess clinical documentation improvement (CDI) programs?

    a. Record review rate

    b. Physician query rate

    c. Record agreement rate

    d. Query agreement rate

437. Which of the following is a good question for a supervisor of coding to ask when evaluating potential fraud or abuse risk areas in the coding area?

    a. Are the assigned codes supported by the health record documentation?

    b. Does the hospital have a compliance plan?

    c. How many claims have not been coded?

    d. Which members of the medical staff have the most admissions to the hospital?

438. The supervisor over the coding division in the HIM department at Community Hospital reviewed the productivity logs of four newly hired coding professionals after their first month. Using the information provided, which employee will require additional assistance in order to meet the standard of 20 medical records coded per day?

Community Hospital Coding Productivity Report Coding Standard: 20 health records per day				
Coder	Week 1	Week 2	Week 3	Week 4
1	90	105	98	107
2	100	105	105	95
3	75	80	85	105
4	80	95	115	110

a. Coder 1

b. Coder 2

c. Coder 3

d. Coder 4

439. Calling out patient names in a physician's office is:

a. An incidental disclosure

b. Not subject to the minimum necessary requirement

c. A disclosure for payment purposes

d. An automatic violation of the HIPAA Privacy Rule

440. The overutilization or inappropriate utilization of services and misuse of resources, typically not a criminal or intentional act is called which of the following?

a. Fraud

b. Abuse

c. Waste

d. Audit

441. The coding staff should be updated at least _____ on compliance requirements.

a. Weekly

b. Monthly

c. Every six months

d. Annually

442. Organizations use of audits in data analysis in order to ensure compliance with policies and procedures is a component of:

a. Internal monitoring

b. Benchmarking

c. Corrective action

d. Educating staff

443. The nursing staff routinely sends text messages to attending physicians to clarify orders during the night shift. The HIM professional should recommend which of the following to refine the policy as the best practice for protecting information that is text messaged?

    a. Send a text message to more than one person.

    b. Enter a person's telephone number each time a text message is sent to him.

    c. Encrypt text messages during transmission.

    d. Presume that telephone numbers stored in memory remain valid.

444. Why is it essential for members of the compliance team to be involved in the entire EHR implementation process?

    a. To ensure HIPAA compliance

    b. To implement external audits

    c. To monitor cut and paste documentation

    d. To mitigate reimbursement risk

445. Which of the following is the process of establishing an organizational culture that promotes the prevention, detection, and resolution of instances of conduct that do not conform to federal, state, or private payer healthcare program requirements or the healthcare organization's ethical and business policies?

    a. Corporate integrity

    b. Meaningful use

    c. Benchmarking

    d. Compliance

446. The Joint Commission is conducting an audit at Community Hospital to determine the hospital's compliance with the Joint Commission standards regarding patient rights. This is an example of a(n):

    a. Complex review

    b. External audit

    c. Internal audit

    d. Casefinding review

447. What is the goal of the clinical documentation improvement (CDI) compliance review?

    a. Compliant MS-DRG assignment between CDI program staff

    b. To ensure corrective action for any compliance concerns

    c. Compliant query generation and physician responses

    d. To ensure compliance between CDI program staff

448. A Recovery Auditing Contractor (RAC) is conducting a review of claims for improper payment at Wildcat Hospital. The review is performed electronically utilizing a software program that analyzes claims data to identify proper payments. This type of review is referred to as a(n):

    a. Automated review

    b. Complex review

    c. Semi-automated review

    d. Semi-complex review

449. What is the most constant threat to health information integrity?

    a. Natural threats

    b. Environmental threats

    c. Internal threats

    d. Human threats

450. Which of the following is the whistleblower provision of the False Claims Act that provides a means for individuals to report healthcare information noncompliance?

    a. *Quid pro quo*

    b. Query

    c. *Qui tam*

    d. Quasi reporting

451. Community Hospital is looking for ways to increase physician referrals. One board member suggested that they offer local physician $100 for every patient referred to the hospital for care. If the hospital goes ahead with the board member's suggestion, what statute is the hospital violating?

    a. Anti-Kickback Statute

    b. False Claims Act

    c. Health Insurance Portability and Accountability Act

    d. Red Flags Rule

452. A postoperative patient was prescribed Lortab prn. Nurse Jones documented in the patient record that she administered one dose of Lortab to the patient, but never actually administered this medication. Nurse Jones then took the Lortab herself. This action would be called?

    a. Drug prescribing

    b. Adverse drug reaction

    c. Sentinel event

    d. Drug diversion

453. Pam is a nursing supervisor in the newborn intensive care unit. During her shift several parents of newborns in the unit are visiting and the neonatologist has also recently been in and has provided orders for several of the newborns. Because of the current workload another nurse in the unit, Jackie, has asked Pam to help her complete the orders. Pam is asked to administer a medication to one of the newborns that Jackie has already retrieved for the patient. Jackie tells Pam that she has double checked the medication both through bar coding and with the order. Before Pam goes to administer the medication, she scans both the medication and the newborn's patient ID band and learns that she has the incorrect medication for this patient. Pam does not administer that medication, but goes back to the order and through the proper steps administers the correct medication. Based on this scenario, which of the following occurred?

   a. Time-out

   b. Serious event

   c. Sentinel event

   d. Near miss

454. Which item below is *not* recommended by the HHS and the OIG for minimum compliance with clinical documentation regulations?

   a. Physicians should include vaccination records

   b. Progress, response, and changes are to be documented

   c. Health record should be completely legible

   d. Past and present diagnosis should be easily accessible

455. Which of the following is an investigational technique that facilitates the identification of the various factors that contribute to a problem?

   a. Affinity grouping

   b. Cause-and-effect diagram

   c. Force-field analysis

   d. Nominal group technique

456. Which of the following groups are included in the feedback loop among denials, management, and clinical documentation improvement (CDI) program staff?

   a. Compliance

   b. Office of the Inspector General

   c. Center for Medicare and Medicaid Services

   d. Payers

457. If a patient receives a _____ from a healthcare organization it indicated that the patient's protected health information was involved in a data breach.

   a. Notice of Breach

   b. Release of Information

   c. Protected Health Breach Notice

   d. Receipt of Breach Notice

458. A patient requested a copy of a payment made by her insurance company for a surgery she had last month. The business office copied the remittance advice (RA) notice the organization received from the insurance company but failed to delete or remove the PHI for 10 other patients listed on the same RA. This is an example of:

    a. Audit control

    b. Ransomware

    c. Retrospective review

    d. Security breach

459. The benefits of a coding compliance plan include the following:

    a. Improving patient care

    b. Identifying those who participate in fraud and abuse

    c. Retention of high standard of coding

    d. Increasing the number of denials of healthcare services reimbursement based on coding errors

460. Sarah, a new graduate of a health information technology program, sits for the registered health information technician (RHIT) exam and fails. She does not want her employer to know she failed and tells her coworkers she passed the examination. Sarah then starts using the RHIT credential after her name in work correspondence. A coworker, Nancy, discovers that Sarah is using the RHIT credential fraudulently and notifies the supervisor, Joan. What is the responsibility of Nancy and Joan in this situation?

    a. Contact AHIMA and report the abuse.

    b. Contact the state licensing division.

    c. Contact the Office of the Inspector General.

    d. Contact the HIT program.

461. Which plan should be devised to respond to issues arising from the clinical documentation improvement (CDI) compliance and operational audit process?

    a. CDI response plan

    b. Quality assurance plan

    c. Point of service plan

    d. Corrective action plan

462. In a recent documentation quality audit, the HIM manager discovered that the orthopedic surgeons have a high rate of noncompliance with history and physical examinations being available in the patient's record prior to surgery. Which of the following is the best action for the HIM manager to take to address this noncompliance issue?

    a. Discuss this issue and the importance of compliance with the chief of surgery.

    b. Report the noncompliance to the OIG.

    c. Post the names of noncompliant physicians on the door of the physician's lounge.

    d. Discuss this issue and the importance compliance with the HIM staff.

463. Clinical documentation improvement staff members must work directly with this department to obtain data about retrospective physician queries:

    a. Coding

    b. Health information management

    c. Compliance

    d. Case management

464. Which information governance principle for healthcare is to create a process for ensuring that all the information meets requirements of appropriate laws, regulations, standards, and organizational policies?

    a. Accountability

    b. Compliance

    c. Integrity

    d. Retention

465. Consider the following statements and identify which one is true of a coding compliance plan.

    a. The coding compliance plan should include expectations for coding quality.

    b. The coding compliance plan should outline the criteria for when unbundling is acceptable.

    c. The coding compliance plan must list the specific healthcare organization coding policies that differ from official coding guidelines.

    d. Providers that have a facility-wide compliance plan do not need a coding compliance plan.

466. How does Medicare or other third-party payers determine whether the patient has medical necessity for the tests, procedures, or treatment billed on a claim form?

    a. Review the procedure codes submitted

    b. Review the revenue codes submitted on the claim

    c. Review the diagnosis codes submitted

    d. Review the charges submitted for each service

Use the following table to answer questions 467 and 468.

General Hospital Chart Analyst Accuracy Report Fiscal Year 20XX				
Analyst	Qtr 1	Qtr 2	Qtr 3	Qtr 4
John	97%	95%	98%	100%
Sue	98%	99%	97%	99%
Cathy	90%	95%	95%	96%
Barb	90%	91%	92%	90%

467. If General Hospital's chart analyst accuracy rate standard is 95% how many of the analysts are in compliance with the standard for all four quarters of the fiscal year?

    a. All four analysts are in compliance with the standard for all quarters.

    b. None of analysts are in compliance with the standard for all quarters.

    c. Two of the analysts are in compliance with the standard for all quarters.

    d. Only one of the analysts are in compliance with the standard for all quarters.

468. In reviewing this chart analyst accuracy report, which analyst should be counseled to improve his or her accuracy to meet the compliance standard due to consistent below standard performance?

    a. Cathy

    b. Barb

    c. John

    d. Sue

469. Community Hospital requires that all patients who present to the emergency department with a suspected acute myocardial infarction (AMI) are expected to receive an EKG within 10 minutes of their arrival. Results of a documentation audit by the HIM analyst showed that of the 56 patients who had a suspected AMI during the last quarter, 32 had an EKG within the specified timeframe for a rate of compliance of 57.1%. Is Community Hospital in compliance with the established standard for EKGs performed in the emergency department for suspected AMIs?

    a. No, because only 57.1% of the suspected AMI patients received an EKG.

    b. Yes, because 57.1% of the suspected AMI patients received an EKG.

    c. No, because 32 patients with suspected AMI received an EKG.

    d. Yes, because only 56 patients presented with AMI.

470. In developing a coding compliance program, which of the following would *not* be ordinarily included as participants in coding compliance education?

    a. Current coding personnel

    b. Medical staff

    c. Newly hired coding personnel

    d. Nursing staff

471. Risk determination considers the factors of:

    a. Likelihood and impact

    b. Risk prioritization and control recommendations

    c. Risk prioritization and impact

    d. Likelihood and control recommendations

472. The cardiology department at University Hospital has been receiving numerous claims denials since January 1st. Upon further review, the claims are being rejected due to coding errors. The HIM supervisor conducts audit of the claims. Which of the following is the most likely reason for the claims denials?

    a. The department did not submit the claims timely.

    b. The department performed less procedures since January 1st.

    c. The department neglected to update the chargemaster with the new CPT codes for this calendar year.

    d. The department hired two new nurses effective January 1st.

473. A patient admitted with COPD exacerbation. H&P notes respiratory distress. Oxygen saturation on admission is 86 percent on room air, respiratory rate of 28, and arterial blood gas (ABG) results of PaO_2 45, $PaCO_2$ 50, pH 7.34, with Bipap and oxygen ordered. The patient has abnormal ABGs and your documentation reflects respiratory distress. If you mean acute respiratory failure, please document on this form or the progress note. Thank you.

This query is:

a. A leading query and is there for not a compliant query

b. Is not necessary in this situation

c. A non-leading query and is therefore a compliant query

d. A leading query and is therefore a compliant query

474. Which of the following is a database of individuals and healthcare organizations that are not permitted to participate in or receive payment from any federal healthcare program due to past healthcare-related crimes they committed against the federal government?

a. Whistleblowers Protection Act

b. Exclusions Program

c. Stark Law Program

d. False Claims Act

475. Which of the following is *not* an element of an effective compliance plan?

a. Education and training of all employees on compliance

b. Follow-up on all potential risk factors that may lead to an investigation

c. Principles of conduct

d. Disciplinary action against individuals reporting suspected fraud

476. The HIM analyst conducts a documentation audit and discovered that a new nurse practitioner is borrowing record entries from another source as well as representing or displaying past documentation as current are examples of a potential breach of:

a. Identification and demographic integrity

b. Authorship integrity

c. Statistical integrity

d. Auditing integrity

477. Using data mining, an RAC makes a claim determination at the system level without a human review of the health record. This type of review is called a(n):

a. Automated review

b. Complex review

c. Detailed review

d. Systematic review

478. The three categories that HHS uses to determine the level of effort put into fraud and abuse prevention include:

    a. Reasonable cause, reasonable diligence, unbundling

    b. Reasonable cause, overpayment, willful neglect

    c. Reasonable cause, noncovered services, overpayment

    d. Reasonable cause, reasonable diligence, willful neglect

479. The health record states, "The patient is taken to the operating room where a midline incision is made in the patient's abdomen. The diaphragm is repaired around the esophagus and the abdomen is closed." The code assigned was: 43332 Repair, paraesophageal hiatal hernia (including fundoplication), via laparotomy, except neonatal: without implantation of mesh or other prosthesis. What vital piece of information would an auditor find missing in the documentation presented?

    a. Whether the hiatal hernia was repaired

    b. Whether mesh was used in the procedure

    c. Whether the patient meets the age requirement

    d. Whether a laparotomy was performed

480. Faced with a high DNFB balance, the HIM director has advised the coding staff to focus on high dollar discharges in order to reduce the DNFB balance. Several days into this strategy change the billing office manager calls asking why there is a reduced number of claims coming through the system to be billed? How did this change in coding strategy affect the revenue cycle workflow?

    a. The change in strategy had no impact on the revenue cycle workflow.

    b. The change in strategy reduced the number of coding professionals who were able to process discharges.

    c. The change in strategy increased the number of discharges, which impacted the revenue cycle workflow.

    d. The change in strategy reduced the number of claims being released for billing and slowed the revenue cycle workflow.

481. A consulting pulmonologist documents pneumonia as an impression based on the chest x-ray. However, the attending physician documents bronchitis throughout the record, including in the discharge summary. The CDI professional documents the following query:

    Query: Do you agree with the pulmonologist's impression that the patient has pneumonia? Please document your response in the health record or below.

    Yes _____

    No _____

    Other _____

    Clinically Undetermined _____

    Name: _____ Date: _____

    This query is:

    a. A noncompliant query

    b. A query that is not necessary in this situation

    c. A leading query

    d. A compliant query

482. Compliance actively prevents:

    a. Upcoding and abuse

    b. Unbundling and fraud

    c. Fraud and abuse

    d. Waste and abuse

483. Which information governance principle for healthcare stipulates that documentation related to an organization's IG initiatives be available to its workforce and other appropriate interested parties?

    a. Accountability

    b. Compliance

    c. Integrity

    d. Transparency

484. An example of fraud is:

    a. Directing others to falsely document or bill

    b. Charging excessively for services or treatments

    c. Billing for unnecessary services or treatments

    d. A pattern of coding errors such as upcoding or unbundling

485. It has been brought to the attention of the release of information supervisor that Dr. Black is intentionally failing to comply with or is acting with indifference to the HIPAA law. Dr. Black is considered to be engaging in:

    a. Fraud

    b. Willful neglect

    c. Abuse

    d. Unreasonable diligence

486. The coding supervisor is auditing the health records coded by a newly hired coding professional for compliance with coding guidelines. Which of the following is an example of upcoding?

    a. Assigning an open procedure when the procedure was actually laparoscopic

    b. Assigning a diagnosis code that that has both the organism and the diagnosis in the same code

    c. Assigning a diagnosis code that supports the procedure code

    d. Assigning procedure codes that are individual tests when a combination code is available

487. When coding for medical necessity, which of the following is *not* considered a factor in defining medical necessity:

    a. The likelihood that a proposed healthcare service will have a reasonable beneficial effect

    b. The concept that procedures are only reimbursed as a covered benefit when they are performed for a specific diagnosis or specified frequency

    c. The designation of present on admission (POA) be established for the principal and secondary diagnosis

    d. The healthcare services and supplies are proven or acknowledged to be effective in the diagnosis, treatment, cure, or relief of a health condition

Domain 6 *Leadership*

488. The HIM supervisor at Community Clinic is developing a staffing schedule for the year. Based on average patient volume, the clinic has 8,000 images to be scanned and indexed each day. The standard for scanning is 1,600 images per hour. The standard for indexing of scanned images is 750 per hour. Given these standards, how many scheduled hours will be required daily to meet the scanning and indexing needs for these images each clinic day?

   a. 6 hours per day

   b. 10 hours per day

   c. 12 hours per day

   d. 16 hours per day

489. The acute-care hospital discharges an average of 55 patients per day. The HIM department is open during normal business hours only. The volume productivity standard is six records per hour when coding 4.5 hours per day. Assuming that standards are met, how many FTE coding professionals does the facility need to have on staff in order to ensure that there is no backlog?

   a. 2.85

   b. 5

   c. 14.26

   d. 27

490. Coding productivity is measured by:

   a. Quantity

   b. Quality

   c. Quantity and quality

   d. Volume

491. Quality standards for coding accuracy should be:

   a. At least 80 percent

   b. At least 90 percent

   c. As close to 100 percent as possible

   d. No specific standards are possible

492. A statement or guideline that directs decision-making or behavior is called a:

   a. Directive

   b. Procedure

   c. Policy

   d. Rule

493. Which statement best describes employees who are covered under the Family and Medical Leave Act of 1993?

    a. Any employee of a public agency or private firm

    b. Employees of a public agency or private firm employing 50 or more employees working in 20 or more weeks of a calendar year

    c. Employees of a public agency or private firm employing 50 or more employees working in 20 or more weeks of a calendar year; eligible employees have worked at least 12 months

    d. Female employees of a public agency or private firm employing 50 or more employees working in 20 or more weeks of a calendar year; eligible employees have worked at least 12 months

494. Community Hospital wants to offer information technology services to City Hospital, another smaller hospital in the area. This arrangement will financially help both institutions. In reviewing the process to establish this arrangement, the CEO asks the HIM director if there are any barriers to establishing this relationship with regard to HIPAA. In this situation, which of the following should the HIM director advise?

    a. There are no barriers prescribed by HIPAA for this arrangement.

    b. Community Hospital needs to expand their organized healthcare arrangement to include the other hospital.

    c. City Hospital should obtain a business associate agreement with Community Hospital.

    d. Community Hospital should obtain a business associate agreement with City Hospital.

495. To date, the HIM department has not charged for copies of records requested by the patient. However, the policy is currently under review for revision. One HIM committee member suggests using the copying fee established by the state. Another committee member thinks that HIPAA will not allow for copying fees. What input should the HIM director provide?

    a. HIPAA does not allow charges for copying of medical records.

    b. Use the state formula because HIPAA allows hospitals to use the state formula.

    c. Base charges on the cost of labor and supplies for copying and postage if copies are mailed while following the state copy fee schedule.

    d. Because HIPAA allows for reasonable and customary charges, charge only for the paper used for copying the records.

496. Identify the example that can be used to justify a policy against using the copy and paste function.

    a. Improves the quality of care

    b. Decreases the chances of fraudulent claims

    c. Provides more detailed documentation

    d. Documentation cannot be used for quality improvement purposes

497. Managing the adoption and implementation of new processes is called:

    a. Management by design

    b. Change management

    c. Process flow implementation

    d. Visioning

498. Which of the following is a data collection tool that records the workflow of current processes?

    a. Flowchart

    b. Force-field analysis

    c. Pareto chart

    d. Scatter diagram

499. As part of the clinic's performance improvement program, an HIM director wants to implement benchmarking for the transcription division at a large physician clinic. The clinic has 21 transcriptionists who average about 140 lines per hour. The transcription unit supports 80 physicians at a cost of 15 cents per line. What should be the first step that the supervisor takes to establish benchmarks for the transcription division?

    a. Clearly define what is to be studied and accomplished by instituting benchmarks.

    b. Hold a meeting with the transcriptionists to announce the benchmark program.

    c. Obtain benchmarks from other institutions.

    d. Hire a consultant to assist with the process.

500. After an outpatient review, individual audit results by the coding professional should become part of the:

    a. Individual employee's performance evaluation

    b. Patient's health record

    c. Coding compliance review summary

    d. Mission of the coding team

501. An HIM director reviews the departmental scanning productivity reports for the past three months and sees that productivity is below that of the national average. Which of the following actions should the director take?

    a. Reduce the salary of the nonproductive workers.

    b. Investigate whether there are factors contributing to the low productivity that are not reflected in the national benchmarks.

    c. Meet with departmental supervisors to discuss the issue.

    d. Assess whether or not the current economy is affecting productivity.

502. Which of the following is one of the four criteria describing the basics of best of practice clinical documentation improvement (CDI) programs?

    a. Intangible best practices in middle revenue cycle

    b. Practices must be central to only one area

    c. Must be supported by research and actual application by multiple healthcare systems

    d. Best practices with high validity are included

503. Performance standards are used to:

    a. Communicate performance expectations

    b. Assign daily work

    c. Describe the elements of a job

    d. Prepare a job advertisement

504. A comprehensive retrospective review should be conducted at least once a year of which aspect of the clinical documentation improvement program?

    a. Proficiency statistics

    b. Compliance issues

    c. All query opportunities

    d. Core key measures

505. A coding supervisor who makes up the weekly work schedule would engage in what type of planning?

    a. Long range

    b. Operational

    c. Tactical

    d. Strategic

506. Which of the following is one of the five best practices for management of financial measures in the CDI program?

    a. Track and report on CC capture rates across the organization and by service

    b. Build relationships with QIO and primary insurers

    c. Publish data to benchmarking organizations

    d. Document corrective actions

507. One of the first steps in this managerial function is to perform an environmental scan of internal organization and external industry. This is which managerial function?

    a. Planning

    b. Organizing

    c. Leading

    d. Controlling

508. The HIM department at Memorial Hospital will install a new computer-assisted coding (CAC) system next month. Meetings were held with all coding professionals so they had input into the process and could address any concerns. HIM managers are working together to ensure the process is as smooth as possible. This is an example of what kind of change?

    a. Emergent

    b. Open-ended

    c. Planned

    d. Strategic

509. Clinical documentation policies and procedures should:

    a. Dictate the practices and procedures for medical treatment

    b. Encompass nationally recognized guidelines

    c. Meet all the requirements of physician leaders

    d. Be created by and specifically for each organization

510. Dr. Jones is the first physician in the practice to adopt a new e-prescribing application. He says he likes to use the latest technologies and be a role model for other physicians. Dr. Jones is at what step in the innovation adoption life cycle?

    a. Early adopter

    b. Early majority

    c. Laggard

    d. Late majority

511. Privacy awareness and training must be provided to all employees in order to prevent privacy breaches. This requirement is covered under which of the following laws?

    a. Civil Rights Act of 1991

    b. Consolidated Omnibus Budget Reconciliation Act

    c. Fair Labor Standards Act

    d. Health Insurance Portability and Accountability Act

512. Before the actual job analysis process begins, an HIM manager must complete which of the following?

    a. Collect primary data to support the job analysis

    b. Execute a workflow analysis

    c. Perform a needs assessment

    d. Write a job description

513. A standard of performance or best practice for a particular process or outcome is called a(n):

    a. Performance measure

    b. Benchmark

    c. Improvement opportunity

    d. Data measure

514. Elizabeth prepares a weekly dashboard report with key performance indicators of the HIM department to send to the chief executive officer. Preparation of this report falls under what managerial function?

    a. Planning

    b. Organizing

    c. Leading

    d. Controlling

515. As the assistant director of the HIM department, Judy is responsible for creating a job description for the new application specialist position. As part of the data collection phase, Judy researches the AHIMA Body of Knowledge to locate similar job descriptions already on file. The Body of Knowledge is what source of data?

    a. Primary

    b. Secondary

    c. Tertiary

    d. The Body of Knowledge should not be used a source of data

516. Which of the following items on Abigail's to do list is most likely to require a critical conversation?

    a. Ask Thomas to act as a coach for the new scanning clerk scheduled to start next week.

    b. Meet with the director for a discussion on whether I should consider going back to school for my master's degree.

    c. Tell Patricia she has been selected for promotion to lead transcriptionist to fill the vacancy left when Sara retired.

    d. Place Daniel on probation due to continuing problems with decreasing coding productivity and coding accuracy.

517. Jane is responsible for developing the positions needed for scanning inactive records in anticipation of EHR implementation. Since she has no scanning experience, Jane called the supervisors of the scanning function at three different facilities to pick their brains regarding scanning jobs. This is an example of what type of data collection in the job analysis process?

    a. Using external sources

    b. Diary method

    c. Observation method

    d. Work imaging

518. Which of the following behaviors is an early indicator of resistance to change that an employee might exhibit when presented with a new project?

    a. Repeatedly asking questions during a department meeting about the new project

    b. Missing planning meetings to determine the implementation schedule for the new project

    c. Reading industry articles on the new project to gain knowledge prior to installation

    d. Volunteering to be on an implementation committee for the new project

519. Kevin is responsible for updating all job descriptions in the HIM department in order to gather information about the data analyst position to establish standards. He spends time interviewing and observing Sophie, who has held this job for three years. What type of study in Kevin conducting on the data analyst position?

    a. Coaching

    b. Recruiting

    c. Work imaging

    d. Job sharing

520. A supervisor wants to determine whether the release-of-information staff members are working at optimal output. Which of the following would be most useful to determine this?

    a. Review work attendance records to see who is absent from work the most.

    b. Walk through the work area at random times of the day to make sure that employees are at their desks and working.

    c. Set productivity standards for the area, and review results on a regular basis.

    d. Determine the backlog of work not performed each day.

521. Charles is a supervisor of the imaging section of the HIM department. In trying to update scanning productivity standards, Charles calls around to other area hospitals to ask what their scanning standards are. This is an example of what source of performance data?

    a. Benchmarking

    b. Job appraisal

    c. Observation

    d. Work sampling

522. Delegation is a skill that managers develop to show employees that they trust them with authority to perform certain projects on their own. Delegation falls under what managerial function?

    a. Planning

    b. Organizing

    c. Leading

    d. Controlling

523. What document outlines the work to be performed by a specific employee or group of employees with the same responsibilities?

    a. Union contract

    b. Policy and procedure manual

    c. Job evaluation

    d. Job description

524. Each year when coding updates are published, Amy plans a face-to-face seminar training program for coding professionals, business office employees, and physician office personnel involved in coding and billing. It generally takes her three weeks to complete the training of all necessary personnel. Which method of employee training is being described?

    a. Self-directed learning

    b. On-the-job training

    c. Classroom-based learning

    d. Online training

525. Which of the following is an alternate work schedule option that has been made possible by the growth and development of technology?

    a. Compressed workweek

    b. Flextime

    c. Open systems

    d. Telecommuting

526. Angela's annual performance appraisal is scheduled for next month. She has been asked by her supervisor to provide the names of two peers and one person in another department with whom she regularly interacts. These individuals will contribute to Angela's evaluation. This is an example of what type of performance appraisal method?

    a. 360 performance appraisal

    b. Critical incident method

    c. Essay evaluation

    d. Graphic rating scale

527. Which of the following would be an indicator of process problems in a health information department?

    a. 5% decline in the number of patients who indicate satisfaction with hospital care

    b. 10% increase in the average length of stay

    c. 15% reduction in bed turnover rate

    d. 18% error rate on abstracting data

528. A tornado touched down in the community and multiple patients were brought to the hospital. The HIM director has asked all department personnel to report to the emergency staging area to help with record management. The HIM director is performing which function of management?

    a. Planning

    b. Organizing

    c. Leading

    d. Controlling

529. A governing principle that describes how a department or an organization is supposed to handle a specific situation or execute a specific process is a:

    a. Position statement

    b. Policy

    c. Procedure

    d. Performance appraisal

530. The HIM supervisor has set a key performance standard for the release of information (ROI) staff related to the time between receipt of a request and when the request is sent to the requestor. This standard is considered the ROI:

    a. Control workflow

    b. Overlap

    c. Duplicate rate

    d. Turnaround time

531. HIM managers set different types of standards to evaluate employee performance for functions such as coding, analysis, and release of information. These standards are called:

    a. Productivity standards

    b. Accreditation standards

    c. Privacy standards

    d. Regulatory standards

532. An effective tool used by project managers to show each phase and the associated tasks of a project, the responsible party for each task, and the time frame required for the tasks is a:

    a. Flowchart

    b. PERT chart

    c. Gantt chart

    d. Pie chart

533. To implement a meaningful consent process at a healthcare organization, consumers would need to be informed of the available possibilities and decisions, its importance in continued treatment, the process of releasing their health information and to whom, and what it means for them. This falls under which of the three key components of a meaningful consent program?

    a. Patient education and engagement

    b. Technology

    c. Law and policy

    d. Identity management

534. Community Hospital recently implemented a fully integrated electronic health record (EHR) system. The process for record analysis will be significantly different with this new system. The process is changing from the hybrid to a fully electronic analysis process. Which of the following should the HIM manager modify to reflect this process change?

    a. Policy

    b. Standard

    c. Procedure

    d. Benchmark

535. One element of Helen's SWOT analysis mentions the hospital across town recently sent all their coding professionals home to work remotely. Currently, all coding done at Helen's hospital is done in-house. In a SWOT analysis, remote coding done by the other hospital would be a(n):

    a. Strength

    b. Weakness

    c. Opportunity

    d. Threat

536. The coding staff at University Hospital has access to the internet for research purposes while performing their job duties. The coding manager has noticed an increase in use and distraction by her coding professionals who are using social media while on the job. In this situation, what should the coding manager develop and use to handle the inappropriate use of the internet by her coding staff?

    a. Policy

    b. Standard

    c. Procedure

    d. Benchmark

537. In all positions it is important to develop requirements for employee success to perform their job. For the release of information technician position, the statement, "apply policies and procedures for disclosure of health information to process requests with 98% accuracy," would be considered a:

    a. Procedure

    b. Mission

    c. Policy

    d. Competency

538. A recent HIM trend is instituting a clinical documentation improvement program. This is not a small undertaking. Which of the following can be used by the HIM manager to assist in measuring whether or not the program is successful?

    a. Dashboard

    b. Policy

    c. Procedure

    d. Benchmark

539. A coding professional with a vision impairment may need additional workspace lighting and a larger computer monitor installed with adjustments to screen contrast and magnification. This would an example of a(n):

    a. Unreasonable accommodation

    b. Essential job function

    c. Reasonable accommodation

    d. Discrimination

540. The HIM manager is also the facility privacy officer. In this role, she is required to provide her expertise regarding HIPAA privacy and security regulations. She oversees initial training of the workforce for the organization. Which of the following is the best setting to accomplish this initial training to ensure all workforce members are trained?

    a. College coursework

    b. New employee orientation

    c. On-the-job training

    d. Local HIM association meeting

541. As an HIM manager, Chelsea documents both positive and negative examples of her employee's work throughout the year. She refers to these examples during annual evaluations. This is an example of what type of performance appraisal method?

    a. 360 performance appraisal

    b. Critical incident method

    c. Essay evaluation

    d. Graphic rating scale

542. As the director of HIM services, Mitch receives a weekly report from his coding supervisor. The report graphically displays inpatient and outpatient coding volume data, employee turnover rates, and the number of claim denials due to coding errors. This snapshot report is called a:

    a. Benchmark report

    b. Budget

    c. Dashboard

    d. Performance appraisal

543. A document that describes the steps involved in performing a specific function is a:

    a. Position statement

    b. Policy

    c. Procedure

    d. Performance appraisal

544. The HIM director conducted an analysis of the coding department that revealed 10 of the coding professionals are credentialed and have at least 10 years of experience. However, the top five coding professionals are leaving their employment within the next three months. This is an example of which type of analysis?

    a. External

    b. Internal

    c. Market

    d. Workflow

545. Which of the following is a written description of an organization's formal position?

    a. Hierarchy chart

    b. Policy

    c. Organizational chart

    d. Procedure

546. In a PERT chart, the path with the greatest total duration time that represents the longest amount of time required to complete the total project is referred to as:

    a. Benchmarking

    b. Due process

    c. Check path

    d. Critical path

547. Joe is a supervisor of the imaging section of the HIM department. In trying to update scanning productivity standards, Joe asked the current scanners to track their tasks on an activity log. Each scanner logs the time it takes to scan a specific amount of records. This is an example of what source of performance data?

    a. Benchmarking

    b. Job appraisal

    c. Observation

    d. Work sampling

548. The physical therapy director wants to know how all the patient information is put into the EHR and contacts the HIM manager for clarification. The HIM manager explains that the information systems of radiology, lab, R-ADT demographic information, and billing each feed their material electronically into the EHR. The information systems of radiology, lab, R-ADT demographic information, and billing in this situation describe the foundation systems that collect administrative and clinical data that make up the EHR and are called the:

    a. Source systems

    b. Connectivity systems

    c. Specialty clinical systems

    d. Smart peripherals

549. Simone, the EHR coordinator, is performing part of the annual review of HIE efficiency. Since there are several new providers in town, she wants to verify the integrity of all authorized health information that is sent and received to various healthcare organizations through the HIE. Identify the principle that Simone is testing that describes the unified and smooth exchange of information among various healthcare providers and information systems and software applications.

    a. Privacy

    b. Confidentiality

    c. Infrastructure

    d. Interoperability

550. The patient experience manager at a local hospital is initiating a PI project to improve overall patient satisfaction for all outpatient departments. This manager is providing the budget for the project as well the vision for change. In this situation, the patient experience manager is considered to have what role in this project:

    a. Team member

    b. Surveyor

    c. Sponsor

    d. Team facilitator

Answer Key

Exam 1 Answers

1. **b** Data standards are the agreed-upon specifications for the values acceptable for specific data fields. Data standards allow healthcare organizations to exchange health information in a format that ensures the data remain comparable. A number of different types of data standards are used in healthcare to capture all of the administrative and clinical data that is needed. Identifying data content requirements for all areas of the organization would be the first step to ensure data content standards are identified, understood, implemented, and managed for the hospital's EHR system (Bowe and Williamson 2020, 383–384).

2. **d** Vocabulary standards are a list or collection of clinical words or phrases with their meanings; also, the set of words used by an individual or group within a particular subject field, such as to provide consistent descriptions of medical terms for an individual's condition in the health record (Sayles and Kavanaugh-Burke 2021, 43–44).

3. **b** Consistency means ensuring the patient data is reliable and the same across the entire patient encounter. In other words, patient data within the record should be the same and should not contradict other data also in the patient record (Brinda 2020, 179).

4. **a** The physical examination represents the physician's assessment of the patient's current health status after evaluating the patient's physical condition. The physician performs the physical examination to ensure appropriate treatment and services are ordered for the patient (Brickner 2020a, 104).

5. **d** The problem-oriented health record is better suited to serve the patient and the end user of the patient's information. The key characteristic of this format is an itemized list of the patient's past and present social, psychological, and health problems (Brickner 2020a, 116–117).

6. **d** The Uniform Hospital Discharge Data Set (UHDDS) data characteristics include patient-specific items on every inpatient (Brinda 2020, 159–160).

7. **c** Clinical laboratory reports should be reviewed to determine if a partial thromboplastin time (PTT) test was performed. Medication Administration Records (MAR) should be reviewed to determine if heparin was given after the PTT test was performed (Brickner 2020a, 106, 108).

8. **b** The master patient index (MPI) is the permanent record of all patients treated at a healthcare facility. It is used by the HIM department to look up patient demographics, dates of care, the patient's health record number, and other information (Sayles 2020b, 70).

9. **a** The consultation report documents the clinical opinion of a physician other than the primary or attending physician. The report is based on the consulting physician's examination of the patient and a review of his or her health record (Brickner 2020a, 109).

10. **a** As the HIM department merges two duplicates together, the source system (laboratory) also must be corrected. This creates new challenges for organizations because merge functionality could be different in each system or module, which in turn creates data redundancy. When duplicates are identified, the department managers need to be notified. Addressing ongoing errors within the MPI means an established quality measurement and maintenance program is crucial to the future of healthcare (Sayles 2020b, 72).

11. **c** The gap analysis process compares omitted clinical information received from external providers with the needed clinical information to make a correct diagnosis. Once complete, the HIM professional would analyze the data and develop a plan for correction (Rossiter 2017, 279).

12. **b** The quantitative analysis or record content review process can be handled in a number of ways. Some acute-care facilities conduct record review on a continuing basis during a patient's hospital stay. Using this method, personnel from the HIM department go to the nursing unit daily (or periodically) to review each patient's record. This type of process is usually referred to as a concurrent review because review occurs concurrently with the patient's stay in the hospital (Sayles 2020b, 76–77).

13. **b** A coding manager or physician champion should present documentation issues to educate the medical staff. General areas of concern regarding documentation should be included (Schraffenberger and Kuehn 2011, 386–387).

14. **c** Administered by the federal government Centers for Medicare and Medicaid Services (CMS), the Medicare Conditions of Participation or Conditions for Coverage apply to a variety of healthcare organizations that participate in the Medicare program. In other words, participating organizations receive federal funds from the Medicare program for services provided to patients and, thus, must follow the Medicare Conditions of Participation (Brickner 2020a, 97).

15. **b** When an incomplete record is not rectified within a specific number of days as indicated in the medical staff rules and regulations, the record is considered to be a delinquent record. The HIM department monitors the delinquent record rate very closely to ensure compliance with accrediting standards (Sayles 2020b, 77).

16. **d** Every participating healthcare organization is subject to a periodic accreditation survey. Surveyors visit each facility and compare its programs, policies, and procedures to a prepublished set of performance standards. A key component of every accreditation survey is a review of the facility's health records. Surveyors review the documentation of patient care services to determine whether the standards for care are being met (Sayles 2020b, 67).

17. **b** Medicare-certified home healthcare uses a standardized patient assessment instrument called the Outcomes and Assessment Information Set (OASIS). OASIS items are components of the comprehensive assessment that is the foundation for the plan of care (Selman-Holman 2017, 345).

18. **c** Licensure is the state's act of granting a healthcare organization or individual practitioner the right to provide healthcare services of a defined scope in a limited geographic area. It is illegal in all 50 states to operate healthcare facilities and practice medicine without a license (Fahrenholz 2017a, 82).

19. **a** A pattern used in electronic health records to capture data in a structured manner is called a template. One benefit of using a template is to ensure data integrity upon data entry (Brickner 2020a, 95).

20. **b** Structured data are data that are able to be read and interpreted by a computer. Examples of structured data include check boxes, drop-down boxes, and radio buttons (Brinda 2020, 180–181).

21. **b** The HIM professional should advise the medical group practice to develop a list of statutes, regulations, rules, and guidelines regarding the release of the health record as the first step in determining the components of the legal health records (Rinehart-Thompson 2017b, 170–171).

22. **a** Health records, x-rays, laboratory reports, consultation reports, and other physical documents relating to the delivery of patient care are owned by the healthcare organization (Rinehart-Thompson 2020a, 234–235).

23. **b** Organizational policy should address how personal health information provided by the patient will or will not be incorporated into the patient's health record. Copies of personal health records (PHRs), created, owned, and managed by the patient, are considered part of the legal health record when the organization uses them to provide treatment; however, the PHR does not replace the legal health record (Fahrenholz 2017c, 57).

24. **b** Organizations should develop and maintain an inventory of all documents and data that could comprise the legal health record, considering all locations in the organization (for example, separate departments or servers) where such information could be housed. Organizations should also carefully consider whether to include data such as pop-up reminders, alerts, and metadata. Metadata are data about data and include information that track actions such as when and by whom a document was accessed or changed (Rinehart-Thompson 2020a, 237).

25. **a** Every healthcare facility should have a clinical forms committee to establish standards for design and to approve new and revised forms. The committee should also have oversight of computer screens and other data capture tools (Sayles 2020b, 79).

26. **a** To correct errors or make changes in the paper health record, a single line should be drawn in ink through the incorrect entry. The word error should be printed at the top of the entry along with a legal signature or initials, date, time, and discipline of the person making the change (Sayles 2020b, 78).

27. **c** In the EHR, the user is able to copy and paste free text from one patient or patient encounter to another. This practice is dangerous as inaccurate information can easily be copied. One of the risks to documentation integrity of using copy functionality includes propagation of false information in the record (Sayles 2020b, 82).

28. **b** A complete medical history documents the patient's current complaints and symptoms and lists his or her past health, personal, and family history. In inpatient care, the health history is usually the responsibility of the attending physician (Brickner 2020a, 104–105).

29. **a** The health record typically begins in patient registration with the capture of patient demographic information. The health record is assigned to new patients during the patient registration process. The HIM department works with patient registration to ensure the quality of the data collected and to correct duplicate and other issues with the MPI (Sayles 2020b, 71–72).

30. **a** Qualitative analysis is about the quality of the documentation including the use of approved abbreviations (Sayles 2020b, 76).

31. **c** The HIPAA Privacy Rule requires the covered entity to have business associate agreements in place with each business associate. This agreement must always include provisions regarding destruction or return of protected health information (PHI) upon termination of a business associate's services. Upon notice of the termination, the covered entity needs to contact the business associate and determine if the entity still retains any protected health information from, or created for, the covered entity. The PHI must be destroyed, returned to the covered entity, or transferred to another business associate. Once the PHI is transferred or destroyed, it is recommended that the covered entity obtain a certification from the business associate that either it has no PHI, or all PHI it had has been destroyed or returned to the covered entity (Thomason 2013, 18).

32. **b** HIPAA allows a covered entity to adopt security protection measures that are appropriate for its organization as long as they meet the minimum HIPAA security standards. Security protections in a large medical facility will be more complex than those implemented in a small group practice (Brickner 2020b, 307).

33. **a** The access controls standard requires implementation of technical procedures to control or limit access to health information. The procedures would be executed through some type of software program. This requirement ensures that individuals are given authorization to access only the data they need to perform their respective jobs (Brickner 2020b, 311).

34. **c** Release of information (ROI), also known as disclosure of health information, is the process of providing PHI access to individuals or entities that are deemed to be authorized to either receive or review it. Protecting the security and privacy of patient information is one of a healthcare organization's top priorities, and the HIM department is usually responsible for determining appropriate access to and ROI from patient health records. Knowledge of state and federal confidentiality laws is critical to the ROI function (Rinehart-Thompson 2020b, 274).

35. **b** Data recovery is the process of recouping lost data or reconciling conflicting data after the system fails. These data may be from events that occurred while the system was down or from backed-up data (Sayles and Kavanaugh-Burke 2021, 293).

36. **a** An audit trail is a software program that tracks every single access or attempted access of data in the information system. It can track when an employee has accessed the system, the actions taken, and how long the employee has been logged into a system (Brickner 2020b, 301).

37. **c** Sometimes HIM professionals are subpoenaed to testify as to the authenticity of the health records by confirming that they were compiled in the normal course of business and have not been altered in any way. A subpoena that is issued to elicit testimony is a *subpoena ad testificandum* (Rinehart-Thompson 2020a, 227).

38. **a** A patient has a right to a notice of privacy practices as defined in the HIPAA Privacy Rule. A healthcare provider has to provide the notice no later than the first service delivery. After that first provision of service, there is no requirement to provide a notice every time a patient receives service (Thomason 2013, 113).

39. **a** The HIPAA Privacy Rule states that the covered entity must provide individuals with their information in the form that is requested by the individuals, if it is readily producible in the requested format. The covered entity can certainly decide, along with the individual, the easiest and least expensive way to provide the copies they request. Per the request of an individual, a covered entity must provide an electronic copy of any and all health information that the covered entity maintains electronically in a designated record set. If a covered entity does not maintain the entire designated record set electronically, there is not a requirement that the covered entity scan paper documents so the documents can be provided in that format (Thomason 2013, 102).

40. **c** Audit trails are usually examined by system administrators who use special analysis software to identify suspicious or abnormal system events or behavior. Because the audit trail maintains a complete log of system activity, it can also be used to help reconstruct how and when an adverse event or failure occurred (Brickner 2020b, 301).

41. **a** Confidentiality refers to the expectation that the personal information shared by an individual with a healthcare provider during the course of care will be used only for its intended purpose (Rinehart-Thompson 2020b, 248).

42. **d** Because minors are, as a general rule, legally incompetent and unable to make decisions regarding the use and disclosure of their own health information, this authority belongs to the minor's parent(s) or legal guardian(s) unless an exception applies. Because privacy, security, and confidentiality of minor records are extremely regulated, HIM professionals should also consult state regulations or legal counsel for specific questions. Generally, only one parent signature is required to authorize the use or disclosure of the minor's PHI (Brodnik 2017b, 342).

43. **b** Emancipated minors generally may authorize the access and disclosure of their own PHI. If the minor is married or previously married, the minor may authorize the disclosure or use of his or her information. If the minor is under the age of 18 and is the parent of a child, the minor may authorize the access and disclosures of his or her own information as well as that of his or her child (Brodnik 2017b, 343).

44. **d** The HIPAA Privacy Rule requires that records be produced within 30 days to a patient or their personal representative, with a one-time extension of an additional 30 days if necessary. If such an additional 30 days is needed, the covered entity must notify the patient in writing of the need for additional time (Thomason 2013, 98).

45. **c** In the context of healthcare, privacy can be defined as the right of individuals to control access to their personal health information (Rinehart-Thompson 2020b, 248).

46. **a** One of the most fundamental terms used in the Privacy Rule is *protected health information* (PHI). The Privacy Rule defines PHI as individually identifiable health information that is transmitted by electronic media, maintained in any electronic medium, or maintained in any other form or medium (Rinehart-Thompson 2020b, 251–252).

47. **a** Original health records may be required by subpoena to be produced in person and the custodian of records is required to authenticate those records through testimony (Rinehart-Thompson 2020a, 228–229).

48. **b** The HIPAA Privacy Rule allows communications to occur for treatment purposes. The preamble repeatedly states the intent of the rule is to not interfere with customary and necessary communications in the healthcare of the individual. Calling out a patient's name in a waiting room, or even on the facility's paging system, is considered an incidental disclosure and, therefore, allowed in the Privacy Rule (Thomason 2013, 37).

49. **a** Establishing access controls is a fundamental security strategy. Basically, the term *access control* means being able to identify which employees should have access to what data. The general practice is that employees should have access only to data they need to do their jobs. For example, an admitting clerk and a healthcare provider would not have access to the same kinds of data (Brickner 2020b, 297–298).

50. **b** The HIM professional must consider multiple factors when developing health record retention policies that determine how long health records are to be kept. These factors include applicable federal and state statutes and regulations; accreditation standards; operational needs of the organization; and the type of organization, thus retention policies differ among healthcare facilities (Rinehart-Thompson 2020a, 237–238).

51. **c** Maintaining some type of accounting procedure for monitoring and tracking PHI disclosures has been a common practice in departments that manage health information. However, the Privacy Rule has a specific standard with respect to such recordkeeping. Disclosures for which an accounting is not required, and which are therefore exempt include some of the following examples: TPO disclosures, pursuant to an authorization, and to meet national security or intelligence requirements. PHI sent to a physician that has not treated the patient would need to be accounted for (Rinehart-Thompson 2017d, 247–248).

52. **c** Physical safeguards refer to the physical protection of information resources from physical damage, loss from natural or other disasters, and theft. This includes protection and monitoring of the workplace, computing facilities, and any type of hardware or supporting information system infrastructure such as wiring closets, cables, and telephone and data lines. To protect from intrusion, there should be proper physical separation from the public. Doors, locks, audible alarms, and cameras should be installed to protect particularly sensitive areas such as data centers (Brickner 2020b, 299–300).

53. **c** All threats can be categorized as either internal threats (threats that originate within an organization) or external threats (threats that originate outside an organization). People are not the only threats to data security. Natural disasters such as earthquakes, tornadoes, floods, and hurricanes can demolish physical facilities and electrical utilities (Brickner 2020b, 290).

54. **a** Not all information must be kept forever. Just as the HIM professional must consider multiple factors when determining retention, many factors must also be taken into consideration with regard to health record destruction. These include applicable federal and state statutes and regulations; accreditation standards; pending or ongoing litigation; storage capabilities; and cost (Rinehart-Thompson 2020a, 238–239).

55. **d** The HIPAA Security Rule requires that access to electronic PHI in information systems is monitored. Included in the same standard is the requirement that covered entities examine the activity using access audit logs. Often they record time stamps that record access and use of the data elements and documents; what was viewed, created, updated, or deleted; the user's identification; the owner of the record; and the physical location on the network where the access occurred. Creation of an account through the patient portal by the patient is appropriate use (Thomason 2013, 177).

56. **a** With appropriate policies and procedures in place, it is the responsibility of the organization and its managers, directors, CSO, and employees with audit responsibilities to review access logs, audit trails, failed logins, and other reports. One type of event that would be a trigger event would include employees viewing records of patients with the same last name or address of the employee (Brickner 2020b, 313).

57. **d** In the "Payments" column, Medicare has the highest payment percentage (42 percent) of any of the payers; therefore, Medicare contributes more to the hospital's overall payments (Williamson 2020, 394).

58. **c** Data about patients can be extracted from individual health records and combined as aggregate data. Aggregate data are used to develop information about groups of patients. For example, data about all patients who suffered an acute myocardial infarction during a specific time period could be collected in a database (Sharp 2020, 199).

59. **c** The Medicare Provider Analysis and Review (MEDPAR) file is made up of acute-care hospital and skilled nursing facility (SNF) claims data for all Medicare claims. The MEDPAR file is frequently used for research on topics such as charges for particular types of care and DRGs. The limitation of the MEDPAR data for research purposes is that the file contains only Medicare patients. Community Hospital is excluding MEDPAR data of those patients with a principal diagnosis of UTI or infectious disease because these would not represent a hospital-acquired condition (HAC) because the patients were admitted with those diagnoses. Community Hospital is looking for comparative secondary diagnosis data of Medicare patients from the MEDPAR file to compare their HAC rate for UTIs to the national average from the MEDPAR data (Gordon, M. L. 2020, 489; Sharp 2020, 211).

60. **b** The median is the midpoint of a frequency distribution. It is the point at which 50 percent of observations fall above and 50 percent fall below. If an even number of observations is in the frequency distribution, the median is the midpoint between the two middle observations. It is found by averaging the two middle scores, (x + y) / 2. In the example, the median is 31.5: ([30 + 33] / 2) (Williamson 2020, 407).

61. **a** A table is an orderly arrangement of values that groups data into rows and columns. Almost any type of quantitative information can be organized into tables. Tables are useful for demonstrating patterns and other kinds of relationships. Tables need headings for columns and rows, and they need to be specific and understandable (Williamson 2020, 393–394).

62. **b** A unit of measure that reflects the services received by one inpatient during a 24-hour period is called an inpatient service day. The number of inpatient service days for a 24-hour period is equal to the daily inpatient census—that is, one service day for each patient treated. The calculation is: [(250 + 30) − 40] + 2 = 242 (McNeill 2020, 436–437).

63. **d** A complete history and physical report represents the attending physician's assessment of the patient's current health status, and accreditation standards require it to be completed within 24 hours of admission. In this case, 191 instances of timely H&Ps out of 200 sampled is 95.5% accuracy. The calculation is (191 / 200) × 100 = 95.5% (Brickner 2020a, 104; McNeill 2020, 433).

64. **a** Abstracting is the process of extracting elements of data from a source document and entering them into an automated system. The purpose of this endeavor is to make those data elements available for later use. After a data element is captured in electronic form, it can be aggregated into a group of data elements to provide information needed by the user (Sayles 2020b, 70).

65. **a** Although sometimes used interchangeably, the terms *data* and *information* do not mean the same thing. Data represent the basic facts about people, processes, measurements, conditions, and so on. They can be collected in the form of dates, numerical measurements and statistics, textual descriptions, checklists, images, and symbols. After data have been collected and analyzed, they are converted into a form that can be used for a specific purpose. This useful form is called information. In other words, data represent facts and information represents meaning (Sayles 2020b, 64).

66. **b** Patient care managers are responsible for the overall evaluation of services rendered for their particular area of responsibility. To identify patterns and trends, they take details from individual health records and put all the information together in one place (Sayles 2020b, 66).

67. **b** Patient care outcomes are reviewed to improve the safety and quality of care as well as to identify issues related to medical necessity for treatment and appropriateness of care. Accrediting and licensing entities expect that healthcare organizations will choose appropriate measures for the services they offer. In this situation is it important to determine whether there was a medical or other reason why patients were not given aspirin within 24 hours of arrival at the hospital. This determination is critical to assess compliance with the quality goal (Shaw and Carter 2019, 160).

68. **d** Performance measurement in healthcare provides an indication of an organization's performance in relation to a specified process or outcome. Healthcare performance improvement philosophies most often focus on measuring performance in the areas of systems, processes, and outcomes. Outcomes should be scrutinized whether they are positive and appropriate or negative and diminishing (Shaw and Carter 2019, 40–41).

69. **a** Sampling is the recording of a smaller subset of observations of the characteristic or parameter, making certain, however, that a sufficient number of observations have been made to predict the overall configuration of the data. In this case, 82 records would be a sufficient number to review for coding quality. The calculation is: $(500 \times 0.05) + (480 \times 0.05) + (300 \times 0.05) + (360 \times 0.05) = 82$ records (Shaw and Carter 2019, 72).

70. **b** A run chart displays data points over a period of time to provide information about performance. The measured points of a process are plotted on a graph at regular time intervals to help team members see whether there are substantial changes in the numbers over time (Carter and Palmer 2020, 560).

71. **d** Derived data consist of factual details aggregated or summarized from a group of health records that provide no means of identifying specific patients. These data should have the same level of confidentiality as the legal health record (Fahrenholz 2017c, 56).

72. **d** Internal users of secondary data are individuals located within the healthcare facility. For example, internal users include medical staff and administrative and management staff. Secondary data enable these users to identify patterns and trends that are helpful in patient care, long-range planning, budgeting, and benchmarking with other facilities (Sharp 2020, 199).

73. **d** After the cases to be included have been determined, the next step is usually case finding. Case finding is a method used to identify the patients who have been seen or treated in the facility for the particular disease or condition of interest to the registry, such as cancer in the case of a cancer registry (Sharp 2020, 201).

74. **c** Healthcare Cost and Utilization Project (HCUP) consists of a set of databases that are unique because they include data on inpatients whose care is paid for by all types of payers, including Medicare, Medicaid, private insurance, self-paying, and uninsured patients. Data elements include demographic information, information on diagnoses and procedures, admission and discharge status, payment sources, total charges, length of stay, and information on the hospital or freestanding ambulatory surgery center (Sharp 2020, 214).

75. **b** All states have a health department with a division that is required to track and record communicable diseases. When a patient is diagnosed with one of the diseases from the health department's communicable disease list, the facility must notify the state public health department (Shaw and Carter 2019, 177). .

76. **b** Since the mean is the average and the value next to the "beginner" under coding professional status is 73.3333, round the value to a whole number and the best answer is 73 (Williamson 2020, 406).

77. **d** Data mapping is a process that allows for connections between two systems. For example, mapping two different coding systems to show the equivalent codes allows for data initially captured for one purpose to be translated and used for another purpose (Brinda 2020, 163–164).

78. **a** The first step in analyzing data is to know your objective or the purpose of the data analysis (Williamson 2020, 413).

79. **b** When the tail is pulled toward the right side, it is called a positively skewed distribution; when the tail is pulled toward the left side of the curve it is called a negatively skewed distribution (Williamson 2020, 410).

80. **d** Prescriptive analytics uses information generated from descriptive and predictive analytics and modelling to determine a strategy for the best outcome and to suggest a course of action to solve a problem (Sayles and Kavanaugh-Burke 2021, 36).

81. **b** Structural metadata is the process of acquiring, storing, manipulating, and displaying data. Data models, such as entity-relationship diagrams (ERD) and dataflow diagrams (DFD) are diagrammatical or graphic tools used to help program the system and to identify areas of inefficiency (Sayles and Kavanaugh-Burke 2021, 42).

82. **d** When the patient checks in, patient registration records demographic information, verifies payment method and insurance coverage, and collects the copayment for the visit. These are front-end processes for the revenue cycle (Gordon, M. L. 2020, 475–476).

83. **c** The accounts not selected for billing report is a daily report used to track the many reasons that accounts may not be ready for billing. This report is also called the discharged, not final billed (DNFB) report. Accounts that have not met all facility-specified criteria for billing are held and reported on this daily tracking list. Some accounts are held because the patient has not signed the consents and authorizations required by the insurer. Still others are not billed because the primary and secondary insurance benefits have not been confirmed (Schraffenberger and Kuehn 2011, 436; AHIMA 2017, 81).

84. **a** The Medicare Outpatient Code Editor (OCE) is a software program designed to process data for the Medicare Hospital Outpatient Payment System pricing and to audit facility claims data. The OCE audits claims for coding and data entry errors. The extensive edits in the OCE are applied to claims, individual diagnoses and procedures, and code sets. The procedure and sex conflict edit occurs when the sex of the patient does not match the sex designated for the procedure code reported (Casto and White 2021, 218–219).

85. **a** When the admission or encounter is for management of dehydration due to the malignancy and only the dehydration is being treated, the dehydration is sequenced first, followed by the code(s) for the malignancy (Schraffenberger and Palkie 2022, 148).

86. **c** To begin the review, the coding supervisor checks the inpatient health record to ensure that the diagnosis billed as principal meets the official Uniform Hospital Discharge Data Set (UHDDS) definition for principal diagnosis. The principal diagnosis must have been a principal reason for admission, and the patient received treatment or evaluation during the stay. When several diagnoses meet all of those requirements, any of them could be selected as the principal diagnosis (Schraffenberger and Kuehn 2011, 315).

87. **b**   Because this patient was seen only in the emergency department, he or she would be classified as an outpatient. Diagnoses documented as "probable," "suspected," "questionable," "rule out," "working diagnosis," or other similar terms in the outpatient setting indicate uncertainty and would not be coded as if existing. Rather, code the condition to the highest degree of certainty for that encounter or visit, such as signs, symptoms, abnormal test results, or other reason for the visit. In this case, unspecified chest pain would be coded (Schraffenberger and Palkie 2022, 105).

88. **d**   A complete replacement of the entire device by the same venous access site is being performed. It is a tunneled catheter inserted within the same venous access point. Code 36582 is the correct code (Smith 2021, 133–135).

89. **b**   No mention is made of biopsy, excision of lesion, or occlusion, so following proper steps for coding in CPT, the correct code is 58670 (Huey 2021, 24).

90. **c**   When subcategory codes are provided, they must be used. Codes are to be assigned to the highest level of specificity based on provider documentation. In this situation, code D23.121 is the most specific code for this diagnosis (Schraffenberger and Palkie 2022, 35, 43–44).

91. **d**   The length of multiple laceration repairs located in the same classification are added together and one code is assigned (Smith 2021, 30–31, 83).

92. **c**   As a result of the disparity in documentation practices by providers, querying has become a common communication and educational method to advocate proper documentation practices. Queries may be made in situations where there are clinical indicators of a diagnosis but no documentation of the condition (Brinda 2020, 186).

93. **a**   Medical necessity is based on the effects of a service for the patient's physical needs and quality of life (Gordon, M. L. 2020, 477).

94. **a**   In the outpatient setting, do not code a diagnosis documented as "probable." Rather, code the conditions to the highest degree of certainty for the encounter (Schraffenberger and Palkie 2022, 105).

95. **b**   In cases of a cesarean delivery, the selection of the principal diagnosis should be the condition established after study that was responsible for the patient's admission. If the patient was admitted with a condition that resulted in the performance of the cesarean procedure, that condition should be selected as the principal diagnosis. If the reason for the admission or encounter was unrelated to the condition resulting in the cesarean delivery, the condition related to the reason for the admission or encounter should be selected as the principal diagnosis even if a cesarean was performed (Schraffenberger and Palkie 2022, 493).

96. **a**   Concurrent coding is the type of coding that takes place in the hospital while the patient is still receiving care (AHIMA 2017, 56).

97. **b**   Focused selections of coded accounts are necessary for deeper understanding of patterns of error or change in high-risk areas or other areas of specific concern, such as a focused audit of cases with no CC/MCC to determine why the case-mix is dropped (Schraffenberger and Kuehn 2011, 271).

98. **c**   Present on admission (POA) is defined as present at the time the order for inpatient admission occurs. Conditions that develop during an outpatient encounter, including emergency department, observation, or outpatient surgery, are considered present on admission. This patient was not admitted with a catheter-associated urinary infection and so that condition cannot be coded as POA. The patient was admitted with symptoms of a stroke and diagnoses of COPD and hypertension. The CVA was documented after admission, but the symptoms of the stroke were POA, so this condition would be coded as POA (Gordon, M. L. 2020, 489).

99. **b**   The root operation extirpation is defined as taking or cutting out solid material from a body part. The matter may have been broken into pieces during the lithotripsy previous to this encounter, but at this time the pieces of the calculus are being removed (Kuehn and Jorwic 2021, 87–88).

100. **b**   The root operation performed was division—cutting into a body part without drawing fluids and/or gases from the body part in order to separate or transect a body part. The intent of the operation was to separate the femur; 0Q860ZZ is the correct code. The Section is Medical and Surgical—character 0; Body System is Lower Bones—character Q; Root Operation is Division—character 8; Body Part is Femur, Right—character 6; Approach is Open—character 0; No Device—character Z; and No Qualifier—character Z (Kuehn and Jorwic 2021, 27–29, 95).

101. **b**   Local coverage determination (LCD) is used to determine coverage on a Medicare Administrative Contractor-wide, intermediary-wide, or carrier-wide basis (rather than nationwide, as with a NCD). LCDs are educational materials that assist facilities and providers with correct billing and claims processing. Within the LCD is a listing of ICD-10-CM codes that indicate what is covered and what is not covered. For example, a procedure may be covered by Medicare, but is not reimbursed by Medicare because it does not meet medical necessity (Casto and White 2021, 215–216).

102. **a**   Medicare severity diagnosis-related group (MS-DRG) sets exist where the listings of diagnoses used to drive the grouping are the same, but the presence or absence of a complication or comorbidity (CC) diagnosis or major complication or comorbidity (MCC) diagnosis assigns the case to a higher or lower MS-DRG. MS-DRG sets may contain two or three MS-DRGs. These MS-DRG relationships and sets pose a compliance concern because the health record documentation used to support the coding of principal diagnosis, complications, and comorbidities may not always be clear or used appropriately by the coding professional (such as undercoding). Therefore, inaccurate coding or incomplete coding can lead to incorrect MS-DRG assignment and thus inappropriate reimbursement and can affect a hospital's case mix. This practice may be considered undercoding (Gordon, M. L. 2020, 493–494).

103. **d**   Medicare does have a provision that a patient may be billed for a test that is not medically necessary if he or she receives an advance beneficiary notice (ABN) before the test is performed. Therefore, not only must the registration staff determine whether the sign or symptom is sufficient, they also may contact the patient's physician to obtain a new order or, if a new order is not provided, to issue an ABN. Success in the patient registration process involves a thoroughly educated staff with the tools to determine medical necessity, the processes in place to clarify orders, and the ability to obtain signatures on ABNs (Schraffenberger and Kuehn 2011, 467).

104. **c**   Front-end utilization management (UM) is essential to the prevention of denials for inappropriate levels of care. UM staff work with the physician to ensure that the requested services meet medical necessity requirements and are provided in the most appropriate setting. When the insurer denies the claim, an appeal may be possible (Schraffenberger and Kuehn 2011, 467).

105. **a**   CDI metrics are key indicators used to monitor the effectiveness of CDI programs. One of the most widely used key indicators for a CDI program is the case-mix index. A strong CDI program will strengthen the case-mix index because the quality and specificity of the documentation help the coding professionals to choose the appropriate codes (Foltz and Lankisch 2020, 521).

106. **d**   Procedure 25500 has a "T" status indicator, which indicates that it is a significant procedure and multiple procedure reductions will apply. In this case, there is only one CPT procedure code that is a status "T" indicator, so 100 percent of the fee-based APC will be paid (Casto and White 2021, 110).

107. **b**   There are two types of transfer cases under the inpatient prospective payment system (IPPS). The first category is a patient transfer between two IPPS hospitals. A type 1 transfer is when a patient is discharged from an acute IPPS hospital (Community Hospital in this case) and is admitted to another acute IPPS hospital (Big Medical Center) on the same day. Payment is altered for the transferring hospital and is based on a per diem rate methodology. The transferring facility receives double the per diem rate for the first day plus the per diem rate for each day thereafter for the patient LOS. The receiving facility receives the full PPS payment rate for the case (Casto and White 2021, 80).

108. **a**   The responsibilities of the quality improvement organizations include reviewing health records to confirm the validity of hospital diagnosis and procedure coding data completeness (Foltz and Lankisch 2020, 508–509).

109. **c**   Charge capture is the accounting for all reportable services and supplies rendered to a patient. There are numerous services and supplies associated with each patient encounter that can be categorized (Casto and White 2021, 142).

110. **b**   A claim denial occurs when an insurance company declines payment for a claim based on a variety of factors. In this situation, there was no code assigned that justified the need for the CT exam. The documentation that justified this exam was included in the record, but missed by the coding professional. In this instance it is appropriate for the code to be added to the claim and the claim to be resubmitted to the payer (Casto and White 2021, 219).

111. **a**   It is common for hospitals and large physician practices to include financial counseling as a service to their patients as they try to manage payment of a deductible while receiving essential healthcare services. This counseling may take many forms including offering payment plans, healthcare loans, or payment support from manufacturers of high-cost pharmaceuticals (Casto and White 2021, 139).

112. **b**   Adjudication is the determination of the reimbursement amount based on the beneficiary's insurance plan benefits. When clean claims are submitted, electronic adjudication can occur. Four outcomes may occur from adjudication: payment, suspend, reject, or deny. If the outcome is payment, then the reimbursement for the claim is paid without review or further processing (Casto and White 2021, 170).

113. **c**   Because the use of a modifier can alter the meaning of the code, it is important that modifiers only be applied to HCPCS codes when documentation in the medical record supports the application of the modifier. Thus, inclusion of modifiers in the CDM is rare, but some facilities do use this practice. CDM teams should pay close attention to modifier reporting guidelines if they choose to include a modifier in the CDM. CDM units should consider all compliance implications that could arise because when included as a line item data element the modifier is reported with the associated HCPCS code every time the charge code is activated (Casto and White 2021, 148–149).

114. **a**   Appointments to the Board of Directors is important information, but the Joint Commission requires detailed information on the responsibilities and actions of the Board, not necessarily its composition. The Joint Commission requires healthcare organizations to collect data on each of these areas: medication management, blood and blood product use, restraint and seclusion use, behavior management and treatment, operative and other invasive procedures, and resuscitation and its outcomes (Shaw and Carter 2019, 304, 313).

115. **b**   One of the elements of the auditing process is identification of risk areas. Selecting the types of cases to review is also important. Examples of various case selection possibilities include chargemaster description for accuracy (Foltz and Lankisch 2020, 513–514; Casto and White 2021, 144).

116. **b**   Coding compliance activities would not include a financial incentive for coding professionals to commit fraud, to code diagnoses and procedures before documentation is complete, or to spend resources reviewing accurately paid claims. Providing a financial incentive to coding professionals for coding claims improperly would be against any coding compliance plan and would also be a violation of AHIMA's Standards of Ethical Coding. One of the basic elements of a coding compliance program includes developing policies and procedures for identifying coding errors (Foltz and Lankisch 2020, 518–519).

117. **a**   The government and other third-party payers are concerned about potential fraud and abuse in claims processing. Therefore, ensuring that bills and claims are accurate and correctly presented is an important focus of healthcare compliance (Foltz and Lankisch 2020, 518–519).

118. **a**   Healthcare fraud is an intended and deliberate deception or misrepresentation by a provider, or by representative of a provider, that results in a false or fictitious claim. These false claims then result in an inappropriate payment by Medicare or other insurers (Foltz and Lankisch 2020, 500).

119. **c**   Ethical coding practices must be followed with appropriate employee counseling and remediation (Foltz and Lankisch 2020, 512–513).

120. **c**   An occurrence report is a structured data collection tool that risk managers use to gather information about potentially compensable events. Effective occurrence reports carefully structure the collection of data, information, and facts in a relatively simple format (Shaw and Carter 2019, 200).

121. **a**   When other healthcare providers provide records, it is done to ensure the continuity of care for the individual. Many covered entities either include the whole file or copies of the file as part of the covered entity's record, with the assumption that the treating physician has used some or all of the records to decide how to treat the patient. Any copies that are included with the records of the individual are, therefore, considered part of the individual's designated record set and should be released (Thomason 2013, 99).

122. **a**   Healthcare fraud is defined as an intentional misrepresentation that an individual knows to be false or does not believe to be true and makes, knowing that the representation could result in some unauthorized benefit to himself or herself or some other person. An example of fraud is billing for a service that was not furnished (Casto and White 2021, 200).

123. **d** Each function should have its own acceptable level of performance and monitoring should be performed to confirm the standards are met. If not, corrective actions should be taken (Sayles 2020b, 79).

124. **b** Reasonable diligence is when the healthcare provider has taken reasonable actions to comply with the legislative requirements (Foltz and Lankisch 2020, 506).

125. **b** Unbundling is the practice of using multiple codes to bill for the various individual steps in a single procedure rather than using a single code that includes all of the steps of the comprehensive procedure code. In this situation, the penalty is the overpayment of the $75 for all 175 claims overpaid as well as three times the total amount of the overpayment (175 × $75 = $13,125 then; $13,125 × 3 = $39,375) (Foltz and Lankisch 2020, 500).

126. **c** The resource that the facility compliance officer should consult to provide information on ongoing reviews and audits each year in programs administered by the department of Health and Human Services (HHS) is the OIG workplan (Casto and White 2021, 201).

127. **c** Hospitals strive to keep incident reports confidential, and in some states incident reports are protected under statutes protecting quality improvement studies and activities. Incident reports themselves should not be considered a part of the health record. Because the staff member mentioned in the record that an incident report was completed, it will likely be discoverable as the health record is already a discoverable document (Fahrenholz 2017a, 89).

128. **d** The purpose of the risk management program is to link risk management functions to related processes of quality assessment and PI. The basic functions of healthcare risk management programs are similar for most organizations and include risk identification and analysis, loss prevention and reduction, and claims management (Carter and Palmer 2020, 572).

129. **a** Treatment, payment, and operations (TPO) is an important concept because the Privacy Rule provides a number of exceptions for PHI used or disclosed for TPO purposes. Treatment means providing, coordinating, or managing healthcare or healthcare-related services by one or more healthcare providers (Rinehart-Thompson 2020b, 253).

130. **b** A cause-and-effect diagram, also known as a fishbone diagram because of its characteristic fish shape, is an investigation technique that facilitates the identification of the various factors that contribute to a problem. It facilitates root-cause analysis in order to determine the cause of the problem (Carter and Palmer 2020, 565).

131. **d** Gaining access to electronic health record systems is a complex challenge in regard to record integrity, information security, linkage of information for continuum of care within different e-health systems, and the development of software for health information management purposes (Hamilton 2020, 674).

132. **d** The supervisor is responsible for ensuring turnaround times are met. Turnaround time is the time between receipt of request and when the information is sent to the requester (Sayles 2020b, 70).

133. **b** An LCD policy contains reasonable and necessary provisions regarding a supply, procedure, or service. For example, a list of codes describing which conditions are a medical necessity and which conditions do not warrant medical necessity may be provided in an LCD policy (Casto and White 2021, 216).

134. **b** Work measurement is based on assessment of internal data collected on actual work performed within the organization and the calculation of time it takes to do the work. Employees log what they do and the time spent on tasks in units of work received and processed each day. 23 charts / 7.5 hours = 3.06, which is rounded to three charts per hour (Prater 2020, 629).

135. **a** The question is asking for the least amount of hours needed to meet the 24-hour turnaround time. The average discharge in a 24-hour period is 120 patients, and the average number of pages for each patient chart is 200. So, 120 × 200 = 24,000 pages in a 24-hour period. Each chart must be prepped, scanned, checked for quality, and indexed. The highest number of pages that can go through all these processes in an hour would be: 500 images in prepping; 2,400 images in scanning; 2,000 images in quality control; and 800 images in indexing.

     - 24,000 / 500 = 48 hours needed for prepping
     - 24,000 / 2,400 = 10 hours for scanning
     - 24,000 / 2,000 = 12 hours for quality control
     - 24,000 / 800 = 30 hours for indexing
     - 48 + 10 + 12 + 30 = 100 hours, at least, needed each day to meet a 24-hour turnaround time (Prater 2020, 628–629).

136. **d** The database management system is the best option to collect, store, manipulate, and retrieve data for this situation. Paper and word-processing documents cannot sort and store the data in a meaningful way for this purpose. Spreadsheets should be used for accounting-type functions and not for data storage (Sayles and Kavanaugh-Burke 2021, 39).

137. **b** Once project planning is completed, execution (or implementation) begins. This is where installation of equipment or construction begins, and any policy or procedure manuals should be prepared for distribution (Shaw and Carter 2019, 370).

138. **a** Interoperability is the ability of different information systems and software applications to communicate and exchange data (Sayles and Kavanaugh-Burke 2021, 198).

139. **a** Current cost: $50 × 40 calls per day = $2,000 per day × 365 days = $730,000. Cost with reduced number of help desk calls: $50 × (40 × 0.80) calls per day = $1,600 per day × 365 days = $584,000, or a savings of $146,000. Training costs of $100,000 will be recouped and a savings of $46,000 realized (Gordon, L. L. 2020a, 541–542).

140. **a** Comparing an organization's performance to the performance of other organizations that provide the same types of services is known as external benchmarking. The other organizations need not be in the same region of the country, but they should be comparable organizations in terms of patient mix and size (Shaw and Carter 2019, 70).

141. **c** Performance standards should be based on both accuracy and volume. In this situation, 114 / 0.60 = 190; 190 − 114 = 76 more pages will need to be indexed to meet the productivity standard (Kelly and Greenstone 2020, 183).

142. **a** Whether selecting a permanent staff team or members of a team for a short-term project, making the right choice is fundamental to the team's success. Putting together a team involves understanding the challenges to be faced and considering all of the perspectives, experience, and knowledge that will be needed. The members of the team should be selected for what they can contribute to the team. Member selection should not be based purely on job title; rather, team members should be selected for the tasks that they actually can perform and the responsibilities they can carry out (Gordon, L. L. 2020b, 596–597).

143. **b** Employee self-appraisal provides the opportunity for the employee to keep the supervisor informed of accomplishments and issues (Prater 2020, 632).

144. **a** Certified EHR technology (CEHRT) is a complete EHR that meets the requirements included in the definition of a qualified EHR and has been tested and certified in accordance with the certification program established by the ONC (Sayles and Kavanaugh-Burke 2021, 203).

145. **d** In parallel work division, the same tasks are handled simultaneously by several workers; each completes all steps in the process from beginning to end, working independently of the other employees (Prater 2020, 625).

146. **d** Reported performance data are regularly analyzed for variance. Variance—where actual performance does not meet, varies, or is significantly different from the standard—should be further assessed (Prater 2020, 630).

147. **c** Speech recognition can be very effective in certain situations when data entry is fairly repetitive and the vocabulary used is fairly limited. As speech recognition improves, it is becoming a replacement for other forms of dictation. In some cases, the user reviews the speech as it is being converted to type and makes any needed corrections; in other cases, the speech is sent to a special device where it generates type for another individual to review and edit (Sayles and Kavanaugh-Burke 2021, 20).

148. **d** The PERT technique provides a structure that requires the project team to identify the order and projected duration of activities needed to complete a project. The most helpful element of PERT is that it identifies those critical activities that must be completed on time in order for the entire project to meet its final deadline (Shaw and Carter 2019, 370).

149. **b** Performance monitoring is data driven. The organization's leadership uses the information displayed on the dashboard to guide operations and determine improvement projects. Having real-time data in an easily assessable format like a dashboard allows leaders to keep track of high-impact, high-risk, or high-value processes and make adjustments on a daily basis if needed (Carter and Palmer 2020, 552).

150. **d** Timeliness of the scanning and quality control processes should be monitored. In this situation, each clinic visit represents a patient record that will need to be scanned and quality control completed. The calculation is: (500 / 50) + (500 / 40) = 22.5 hours per day (White 2020, 156; Prater 2020, 628–629).

Exam 2 Answers

1. **c** Policies and procedures need to be in place to address amendments and corrections in the EHR. In the event that an amendment, addendum, or deletion needs to be made the EHR should retain the previous version of the document and identify who made the change along with the date and time that the change was made (Sayles 2020b, 83).

2. **b** A do-not-resuscitate order is a physician's order documenting a patient's (or a substitute decision maker's) desire for no desired resuscitation attempts. Although a DNR order results from a desire expressed in an advanced directive, it does not replace the need for that directive. The health record should contain documentation indicating the presence of a DNR order (Selman-Holman 2017, 377).

3. **a** Any surgical procedure requires special documentation. The entire process is recorded with an anesthesia report, operative report, and recovery room report (Brickner 2020a, 108–109).

4. **d** Because the ability to manipulate the data is reduced, it is recommended that little, if any, free text is used (Sayles 2020b, 82).

5. **a** Data precision is the term used to describe expected data values. As part of data definition, the acceptable values or value ranges for each data element must be defined. For example, a precise data definition related to gender would include three values: male, female, and unknown (Brinda 2020, 180).

6. **b** Cancer registries are typically maintained by hospitals on a voluntary basis or as mandated by state law. Many states require that hospitals report their data to a central statewide registry or incidence surveillance program (Sharp 2020, 202).

7. **c** The operative report describes the surgical procedures performed on the patient. Each report typically includes the name of the surgeon and assistants; date, duration, and description of the procedure; preoperative and postoperative diagnosis; estimated blood loss; descriptions of any unusual or unique events during the course of the surgery, normal and abnormal findings, as well as any specimens that were removed (Brickner 2020a, 108–109).

8. **d** Structured data are required for a CDS system; hence, templates guide collection of the structured data. Digital dictation and scanned images do not yield structured data for subsequent processing in a CDS system. Alerting programs are one of (many) functions of a CDS system (Bowe and Williamson 2020, 368–369).

9. **a** If missing or incomplete information is identified during record analysis, HIM personnel can issue deficiency notification(s) to the appropriate caregiver to assure the completeness of the health record. An addendum is a supplement to a signed report that provides additional health information within the health record. In this type of correction, a previous entry has been made and the addendum provides additional information to address a specific situation or incident (Sayles 2020b, 78).

10. **a** Data Elements for Emergency Department Systems (DEEDS) is a data set to support the uniform collection of data in hospital-based emergency departments and to reduce incompatibilities in emergency department records. Because DEEDS is based on emergency department records it would be helpful in developing a trauma registry (Brinda 2020, 156).

11. **d** Review of body systems is typically documented in the report of a physical examination. This would include documentation regarding the HEENT (head, eyes, ears, nose, and throat) and the chest (Brickner 2020a, 104–106).

12. **b** Error management is part of data integrity which means that data should be complete, accurate, consistent, and up-to-date. Ensuring the integrity of healthcare data is important because providers use data in making decisions about patient care (Johns 2015, 211).

13. **c** Standardization of the collection of patient data is essential to collect the proper information and reach data quality levels needed to support the enhancement of patient care and the healthcare industry. Templates can be created for common types of notes, visits, and procedures (Brinda 2020, 180–181).

14. **a** The EMPI is a list or database created or maintained by a healthcare facility to record the name and identification number of every patient and activity that has ever been admitted or treated in the facility. When a healthcare enterprise is more than one facility and the patient is seen at two or more places, the enterprise master patient index (EMPI) links the patient's information at the different facilities (Sayles 2020b, 71).

15. **b** Templates are a cross between free text and structured data entry. The user is able to pick and choose data that are entered frequently, thus requiring the entry of data that change from patient to patient. Templates can be customized to meet the needs of the organization as data needs change by physician specialty, patient type (surgical/medical/newborn), disease, and other classification of patients. In this situation a template would provide structured data entry for the admission date (Sayles and Kavanaugh-Burke 2021, 217).

16. **d** Demographic data is used to identify an individual, such as name, address, gender, age, and other information linked to a specific person (Gordon, M. L. 2020, 474).

17. **a** A data dictionary is a descriptive list of the data elements to be collected in an information system or database whose purpose is to ensure consistency of terminology (Brinda 2020, 155–156).

18. **c** Edit checks assist in ensuring data integrity by allowing only reasonable and predetermined values to be entered into the computer (Brickner 2020b, 301).

19. **d** Characteristics for data entry should be uniform throughout the health record to ensure consistency. Data must have definitions and be uniform to prevent information inconsistencies (Sayles and Kavanaugh-Burke 2021, 25).

20. **c** Reviewing for deficiencies is an example of quantitative analysis. The goal of quantitative analysis is to make sure there are no missing reports, forms, or required signatures in a patient record. Timely completion of this process ensures a complete health record (Sayles 2020b, 76–77).

21. **b** The credentialing and privileging process for the initial appointment and reappointment of independent practitioners should be defined in the healthcare organization's medical staff bylaws and should be uniformly applied (Shaw and Carter 2019, 279).

22. **d** One of the major purposes of a health record is to serve as the legal business record of an organization and as evidence in lawsuits or other legal actions, and as such, it would be the record released upon a valid request (Rinehart-Thompson 2017b, 170–171).

23. **a** An advanced directive is a written document that provides directions about a patient's desires in relation to care decisions for use by healthcare workers if the patient is incapacitated or not capable of communication. Physician orders for do not resuscitate (DNR) should be consistent with the patient's advanced directives (Selman-Holman 2017, 377).

24. **a** In the EHR, the user is able to copy and paste free text from one patient or patient encounter to another. This practice is dangerous as inaccurate information can easily be copied. One of the risks to documentation integrity of using copy functionality includes the inability to identify the author of the documentation (Sayles 2020b, 82).

25. **d** The tool that Clara is using is a personal health record. An individual can use a personal health records to collect, track, and share past and current information about his or her health (Sayles 2020b, 88).

26. **b** The health record may have multiple versions of the same document; for example, a signed and an unsigned copy of a document. To address the issues that result from having multiple versions of the same document, policies and procedures addressing version control must be developed (Sayles 2020b, 81–82).

27. **c** Administrative data describes patient identification, diagnosis, procedures, and insurance. Patient registration information would be considered administrative data as would patient account information. A significant portion of administrative data is demographic data (Brickner 2020a, 110).

28. **a** Information assets refer to the information collected during day-to-day operations of a healthcare organization that has value within an organization. For example, patient data collected to support patient care is an example of information assets for the organization (Brinda 2020, 166).

29. **c** Data integrity is the assurance that the data entered into an electronic system or maintained on paper are only accessed and amended by individuals with the authority to do so. Data integrity includes data governance, patient identification, authorship validation, amendments and record correction, and audit validation for reimbursement purposes. These functions ensure that the data is protected and altered by authorized individuals as per policy. Assuring documentation that is being changed is permanently deleted from the record would not be a guideline for maintaining the integrity of the health record (Brinda 2020, 172–173).

30. **c** Policies and procedures need to be in place to address amendments and corrections in the EHR. In the event that an amendment, addendum, or deletion needs to be made the EHR should retain the previous version of the document and identify who made the change along with the date and time that the change was made (Sayles 2020b, 81–82).

31. **b** Device and media controls require the facility to specify proper use of electronic media and devices (external drives, backup devices, and such). Included in this requirement are controls and procedures regarding the receipt and removal of electronic media that contain protected health information and the movement of such data within the facility. The entity must also address procedures for the transfer, removal, or disposal—including reuse or redeployment—of electronic media (Brickner 2020b, 310).

32. **b** An issue with the quality of the MPI is an overlay, where a patient is erroneously assigned another person's health record number. When this happens, patient information from both patients becomes commingled and care providers may make medical decisions based on erroneous information, increasing the legal risks to the healthcare organization and quality of care risks to the patient as well (Sayles 2020b, 72).

33. a   Audit trails are a recording of activities occurring in an information system. Audit trails can monitor system level controls such as log-in, log-out, unsuccessful log-ins, print, query, and other actions. It also records user-identification information and the date and time of the activity. Audits should be scheduled periodically, but can also be performed when a problem is suspected (Sayles and Kavanaugh-Burke 2021, 297–298).

34. a   Health record retention policies depend on a number of factors. They must comply with state and federal statutes and regulations. Retention regulations vary by state and possibly by organization type. Health records should be retained for at least the period specified by the state's statute of limitations for malpractice, and other claims must be taken into consideration when determining the length of time to retain records as evidence (Rinehart-Thompson 2020a, 237).

35. d   In the HIPAA Security Rule, one of the technical safeguards standards is access control. This includes automatic log-off, which ensures processes that terminate an electronic session after a predetermined time of inactivity (Reynolds and Brodnik 2017, 277).

36. a   In order to maintain patient privacy certain audits may need to be completed daily. If a high-profile patient is currently in a facility, for example, access logs may need to be checked daily to determine whether all access to this patient's information by workforce is appropriate (Thomason 2013, 173).

37. c   The HIPAA Privacy Rule permits healthcare providers to access protected health information for treatment purposes. However, there is also a requirement that the covered entity provide reasonable safeguards to protect the information. These requirements are not easy to meet when the access is from an unsecured location, although policies, medical staff bylaws, confidentiality or other agreements, and a careful use of new technology can mitigate some risks (Thomason 2013, 46).

38. b   Associated with ownership of health records is the legal concept of the custodian of records. The custodian of health records is the individual who has been designated as having responsibility for the care, custody, control, and proper safekeeping and disclosure of health records (Brodnik 2017a, 9).

39. a   If the paper health record is destroyed, the imaging record would be the legal health record. This may not be the case if the paper record is retained. State laws typically view the original health record as the legal record when it is available. Those who choose to destroy the original health record may do so within weeks, months, or years of scanning. If the record was destroyed according to guidelines for destruction and no scanned record exists, the certificate of destruction should be presented in lieu of the record (Rinehart-Thompson 2017b, 197–199).

40. c   A firewall is a part of a computer system or network that is designed to block unauthorized access while permitting authorized communications. It is a software program or device that filters information between two networks, usually between a private network like an intranet and a public network like the internet (Brickner 2020b, 301).

41. d   A subpoena *duces tecum* instructs the recipient to bring documents and other records with himself or herself to a deposition or to court (Rinehart-Thompson 2017a, 59).

42. b   There are three exceptions to a breach. All of these answers fall into one of these categories with the exception of the records sent to the patient's attorney. He does not work for the covered entity and an authorization is required (Rinehart-Thompson 2020b, 270).

43. **b** Beneficence would require the HIM professional to ensure that the information is released only to individuals who need it to do something that will benefit the patient (for example, to an insurance company for payment of a claim) (Hamilton 2020, 656).

44. **c** Privacy, confidentiality, and security are related, but distinct, concepts. In the context of healthcare, privacy can be defined as the right of individuals to control access to their personal health information. Confidentiality refers to the expectation that the personal information shared by an individual with a healthcare provider during the course of care will be used only for its intended purpose. Security is the protection of the privacy of individuals and the confidentiality of health records (Johns 2015, 210–211).

45. **a** If physicians were to dictate information regarding patients they are treating in the facility, the disclosure of protected health information within the voice recognition system would be considered healthcare operations and, therefore, permitted under the HIPAA Privacy Rule. If physicians, who are separate covered entities, are dictating information on their private patients, however, it would be necessary for physicians to obtain a business associate agreement with the facility. It is permitted by the Privacy Rule for one covered entity to be a business associate of another covered entity (Thomason 2013, 26).

46. **a** Files of patients who have not been at the facility for a specified period, may be purged or removed and sent to the storage facility (Sayles 2020b, 74).

47. **b** Data integrity means that data should be complete, accurate, consistent, and up-to-date. With respect to data security, organizations must put protections in place so that no one may alter or dispose of data in a manner inconsistent with acceptable business and legal rules (Johns 2015, 211).

48. **c** To preserve discoverable data, they must also ensure that records involved in litigation or potential litigation are preserved through a legal hold, which is generally a court order to preserve a health record if there is concern about destruction. A legal hold supersedes routine destruction procedures. It also prevents spoliation—the act of destroying, changing, or hiding evidence intentionally (Rinehart-Thompson 2020a, 228).

49. **a** A security threat is anything that can exploit a security vulnerability. Vulnerability is a weakness or gap in security protection. In this situation the lack of encryption for the laptop would be considered a security vulnerability as the contents could be more easily accessed (Johns 2015, 219).

50. **a** HIPAA gives individuals the right to request access to their PHI, but the covered entity may require that requests be in writing. HIPAA allows a reasonable cost-based fee when the individual requests a copy of PHI or agrees to accept summary or explanatory information (Rinehart-Thompson 2020b, 255).

51. **c** There are circumstances where PHI can be used or disclosed without the individual's authorization and without granting the individual the opportunity to agree or object. Some of these circumstances include preventing or controlling diseases, injuries, and disabilities, and reporting disease, injury, and vital events such as births and deaths (Rinehart-Thompson 2020b, 265–268).

52. **c** Breaches by covered entities and business associates (both governed by HHS breach notification regulations) are deemed discovered when the breach is first known or reasonably should have been known. All individuals whose information has been breached must be notified without unreasonable delay, and within 60 days, by first-class mail or a faster method, such as by telephone, if there is the potential for imminent misuse (Rinehart-Thompson 2020b, 271).

53. **a** Every member of the covered entity's workforce must be trained in PHI policies and procedures to maintain the privacy of patient information, uphold individual rights guaranteed by the Privacy Rule, and report alleged breaches and other Privacy Rule violations (Rinehart-Thompson 2020b, 273).

54. **d** Record retention should only be done in accordance with federal and state law and written retention and destruction policies of the organization. AHIMA's recommended retention standards for the master patient index (MPI) is permanent retention (Fahrenholz 2017b, 122).

55. **a** Individuals who are notified that their PHI has been breached must be given a description of what occurred (including date of breach and date that breach was discovered); the types of unsecured PHI that were involved (such as name, Social Security number, date of birth, home address, account number); steps that the individual may take to protect himself or herself; what the entity is doing to investigate, mitigate, and prevent future occurrences; and contact information for the individual to ask questions and receive updates (Rinehart-Thompson 2020b, 271).

56. **d** The process for expert determination of deidentification has four recommended steps. Step 1: The facility should choose the expert for the deidentification analysis. Step 2: Determine the statistical and scientific method to be used to determine the risk of reidentification. Step 3: The expert applies the method to the deidentified data. Step 4: Analyze and assess the risk to the deidentified data (Marc and Sandefer 2016, 22–23).

57. **d** Several factors must be addressed when assessing data quality. These include data accuracy, consistency, comprehensiveness, and timeliness. Cost to process the data does not influence the quality (Brinda 2020, 176–180).

58. **c** Indexing in the EHR can be checked by conducting a random audit. To conduct a study, a subsection of the EHR reports can be checked for mislabeled reports. Any mislabeled reports that are found are noted, and an accuracy rate can be determined and compared against the established standard. In this scenario, there was a 4 percent error rate for the 100 records in the sample. If the cost of each misfile is $200, this would cost the facility $800 ($100 \times 0.04$) $\times$ $200 = $800 (White 2020, 156).

59. **b** The average length of stay is the mean length of stay of hospital inpatients discharged during a given period of time. Add the total days for each patient (for a total of 54 days) and divide by nine patients = six days (McNeill 2020, 441).

60. **c** A line graph may be used to display time trends. A line graph is especially useful for plotting a large number of observations. It also allows several sets of data to be presented on one graph (Williamson 2020, 398).

61. **d** The average daily census is the average number of inpatients treated during a given period of time. There are 30 days in September, so 3,000 / 30 = 100 (McNeill 2020, 437).

62. **a** The number of records per FTE is 2 (number of records per hour) $\times$ 2,080 = 4,160. Therefore, three employees per year are required: 12,500 / 4,160 = 3.0 (Prater 2020, 626).

63. **b** The denominator (the number of times an event could have occurred) in this case would be 263 as 263 women delivered (McNeill 2020, 434).

64. a   In the context of healthcare, demographic information includes the following elements: patient's full name; patient's facility identification or account number; patient's address; patient's telephone number; patient's date and place of birth; patient's gender; patient's race or ethnic origin; patient's marital status; name and address of patient's next of kin; date and time of admission; hospital's name, address, and telephone number (Sayles 2020b, 70).

65. a   A check sheet is used to gather data based on sample observations in order to detect patterns. When preparing to collect data, a team should consider the four *W* questions: *Who* will collect the data? *What* data will be collected? *Where* will the data be collected? *When* will the data be collected? (Shaw and Carter 2019, 72–73).

66. a   A benchmark is a systematic comparison of one organization's measurement characteristics to those of another similar organization. When an organization compares its current performance to its own internal historical data, or uses data from similar external organizations, it helps establish an organization benchmark (Carter and Palmer 2020, 558).

67. c   Once a benchmark for each performance measure is determined, analyzing data collection results becomes more meaningful. Often, further study or more focused data collection on a performance measure is triggered when data collection results fall outside the established benchmark. When variation is discovered or when unexpected events suggest performance problems, members of the organization may decide there is an opportunity for improvement (Shaw and Carter 2019, 27).

68. b   Public health and research uses data in the health record for many reasons including monitoring disease outbreaks (Sayles 2020b, 65).

69. a   A disease index is a listing in diagnosis code number order for patients discharged from the facility during a particular time period (Sharp 2020, 200–201).

70. d   Hospitals set completion standards based on this requirement. Record completion would include the discharge summary $(137 / 150) \times 100 = 91.3\%$ (McNeill 2020, 433).

71. b   The MEDPAR file is frequently used for research on topics such as charges for particular types of care and MS-DRGs. The limitation of the MEDPAR data for research purposes is that the file contains only Medicare patients (Sharp 2020, 211).

72. d   The normal distribution is where data follows a symmetrical curve. The normal distribution is actually a theoretical family of distributions that may have any mean or any standard deviation. In a normal distribution, the mean, median, and mode are equal (Williamson 2020, 408–409).

73. c   The scatter chart is showing a strong positive relationship between age and income because as age increases so does income. A negative relationship would show that as age increases income decreases, and that is not the case in this scatter chart example (Williamson 2020, 399–401).

74. b   It is a requirement of the HIPAA Security Rule to implement ways that document access to information systems that contain electronic PHI. One of the ways to do this is to review the individuals that have viewed, created, updated, or deleted information within a health record. In this instance, the privacy officer should review this information to determine if the patient complaint is valid (Thomason 2013, 177).

75. c Sometimes the organizational characteristic or parameter about which data are being collected occurs too frequently to measure every occurrence. In this case, those collecting the data might want to use sampling techniques. Sampling is the recording of a smaller subset of observations of the characteristic or parameter, making certain, however, that a sufficient number of observations have been made to predict the overall configuration of the data (Shaw and Carter 2019, 72).

76. d A heat map plots all data points as a cell for two given variables or interest, and depending on frequency of observations in each cell, provides color to visualize high or low frequency (Marc and Sandefer 2016, 41).

77. a Data mining is the process of extracting and analyzing large volumes of data from a database for the purpose of identifying hidden and sometimes subtle relationships or patterns and using those relationships to predict behaviors (Bowe and Williamson 2020, 369).

78. b In this example, DNFB met the benchmark in January, February, and June, which is 3/6 or 50 percent of the time (Shaw and Carter 2019, 26–27).

79. b Aggregate data is data extracted from individual health records and combined to form deidentified information about groups of patients that can be compared and analyzed (Sayles 2020b, 66).

80. c Predictive analytics is a process to identify patterns that can be used to predict the odds of a particular outcome based upon observed, historical data—think of the daily weather forecast. Predictive analytics can forecast the hospitalization rate and ventilator demand to help healthcare organizations prepare for the increase in admissions (Sayles and Kavanaugh-Burke 2021, 36).

81. c Administrative metadata is programmed in the information system in order to generate data about the usage of the information system, such as audit trail and activity reports. Administrative metadata also includes decision support functions wherein the information system assists in helping to assemble, manipulate, and prioritize data and make recommendations about specific courses of action that can be taken to address an identified issue (Sayles and Kavanaugh-Burke 2021, 42).

82. d A hospital can monitor its performance under the MS-DRG system by monitoring its case-mix index (CMI). The CMI is the average of the relative MS-DRG weights of all cases treated at a given hospital. The CMI can be used to make comparisons between hospitals and to assess the quality of documentation and coding at a particular hospital (Gordon, M. L. 2020, 493–494).

83. c A comorbidity is a medical condition that coexists with the primary cause of the hospitalization and affects the patient's treatment and length of stay (Schraffenberger and Palkie 2022, 93).

84. a Resolving failed edits is one of many duties of the health information management (HIM) department. Various hospital departments depend on the coding expertise of HIM professionals to avoid incorrect coding and potential compliance issues (Casto and White 2021, 167–168).

85. a CHF is the principal diagnosis and must be sequenced first as shortness of breath is a symptom of CHF, and the respiratory failure is a result of the CHF. The principal diagnosis is the reason for the admission to the hospital after study (Schraffenberger and Palkie 2022, 95).

86. **b** Though the term *valvuloplasty* in the Index leads to Repair, Replacement, or Supplement, this procedure was performed as a percutaneous Dilation. The root operation Dilation is expanding an orifice or the lumen of a tubular body part (Kuehn and Jorwic 2021, 109).

87. **b** The HIM department can plan focused review based on specific problem areas after the initial baseline review has been completed (Schraffenberger and Kuehn 2011, 314–315).

88. **a** This is an example of a circumstance in which the chronic condition must be verified. All secondary conditions must match the definition in the UHDDS for a secondary diagnosis, and whether the COPD does is not clear so the provider should be queried (Schraffenberger and Palkie 2022, 100–101; Brinda 2020, 186–187).

89. **a** The patient has esophageal reflux with no esophagitis mentioned, so K21.9 is the correct diagnosis code. For the ICD-10-PCS procedure code, a closed biopsy of the esophagus was performed via esophagoscopy, so 0DB58ZX is the correct code. The Section is Medical and Surgical—character 0; Body System is Gastrointestinal—character D; Root Operation is Excision—character B; Body Part is Esophagus—character 5; Approach—Via Natural or Artificial Opening Endoscopic—character 8; No Device—character Z; and the procedure was for diagnostic reasons (biopsy)—character X (Schraffenberger and Palkie 2022, 43–44; Kuehn and Jorwic 2021, 27–29, 72–73).

90. **b** The bursitis was the result of the previous crush injury and should be coded as sequela with the seventh character coded as "S" for sequela. The code for the left knee is also used to identify laterality (Schraffenberger and Palkie 2022, 649–650).

91. **a** The health information manager must continuously promote complete, accurate, and timely documentation to ensure appropriate coding, billing, and reimbursement. This requires a close working relationship with the medical staff, perhaps through the use of a physician champion. Physician champions assist in educating medical staff members on documentation needed for accurate billing. The medical staff is more likely to listen to a peer than to a facility employee, especially when the topic is documentation needed to ensure appropriate reimbursement (Hess 2015, 123).

92. **c** Colonoscopy includes examining the transverse colon. Proctosigmoidoscopy involves examining the rectum and sigmoid colon. Sigmoidoscopy involves examining the rectum, sigmoid colon, and may include portions of the descending colon (Smith 2021, 142).

93. **c** Each HCPCS code is assigned to one and only one ambulatory payment classification (APC). The APC assignment for a procedure or services does not change based on the patient's medical condition or the severity of illness. There may be an unlimited number of APCs per encounter for a single patient. The number of APC assignments is based on the number of reimbursable procedures or services provided for that patient. In this instance, the patient has five APCs (Casto and White 2021, 109).

94. **d** The weight of each diagnosis-related group (DRG) is multiplied by the number of discharges for that DRG to arrive at the total weight for each DRG—in this situation 15,192. The total weights are summed and divided by the number of total discharges to arrive at the case-mix index for a hospital: 15,192 / 10,471 = 1.45 (McNeill 2020, 451–452).

95. **d** Hematuria is an adverse effect as opposed to a poisoning because it was correctly prescribed and correctly taken (Schraffenberger and Palkie 2022, 620–621).

96. **c** Begin with the main term of Hernia repair; incisional. The fact that the hernia is recurrent, done via a laparoscope, and is reducible makes the answer 49656. Notice that the use of mesh is included in the code (Huey 2021, 24, 152).

97. **b** Placenta previa is the reason for the C-section and therefore is the principal diagnosis (Schraffenberger and Palkie 2022, 493).

98. **a** When an admission or encounter is for the management of anemia associated with the malignancy, and the treatment is only for anemia, the appropriate code for the malignancy is sequenced first as the principal or first-listed diagnosis followed by the appropriate code for the anemia (such as D63.0, Anemia in neoplastic disease) according to ICD-10-CM Coding Guideline I.C.2.c.1 (Schraffenberger and Palkie 2022, 147–148).

99. **c** The hospital-acquired conditions (HAC) provision is an additional component of pay-for-performance utilizing reported ICD-10-CM diagnosis codes and the present-on-admission (POA) indicator to identify quality issues. A Stage III or IV pressure ulcer not present on admission or identified with the POA indicator on the claim would not be paid for as a CC or MCC because it would be considered an HAC (Casto and White 2021, 85–86).

100. **c** MS-DRG 193 has the highest weight and therefore would have the highest payment (Casto and White 2021, 73–74).

101. **a** The outpatient code editor (OCE) is a software program that applies a set of logical rules to determine whether various combinations of codes are correct and appropriately represent the services provided (Casto and White 2021, 217–218).

102. **b** As a result of the disparity in documentation practices by providers, querying has become a common communication and educational method to advocate proper documentation practices. Queries can be made in situations when there is clinical evidence for a higher degree of specificity or severity (Brinda 2020, 186).

103. **d** Unbundling occurs when individual components of a complete procedure or service are billed separately instead of using a combination code (Bowman 2017, 440).

104. **a** Utilization controls include the prospective and retrospective review of the healthcare services planned for, or provided to, patients. For example, a prospective utilization review of a plan to hospitalize a patient for minor surgery might determine that surgery could be safely performed less expensively in an outpatient setting. Prospective utilization review—often called precertification—is done in managed fee-for-service reimbursement (Gordon, M. L. 2020, 490).

105. **b** The accounts not selected for billing report is a daily report used to track the many reasons that accounts may not be ready for billing. This report is also called the discharged, not final billed (DNFB) report. Accounts that have not met all facility-specified criteria for billing are held and reported on this daily tracking list (Schraffenberger and Kuehn 2011, 436).

106. **a** An appeal is a request for reconsideration of denial of coverage for healthcare services or rejection of a claim. The appeals section of a policy describes the steps the beneficiary must take to appeal a decision about coverage or payment of a claim. Typically, the appeal must be in writing and within a specific time frame of the health insurance company's decision concerning the issue (Casto and White 2021, 25).

107. d Coding errors can affect the Medicare severity diagnosis-related group (MS-DRG) assignment, thus impacting the revenue cycle. Ultimately, the coding supervisor should determine whether the frequency of errors identified demonstrates a trend (Schraffenberger and Kuehn 2011, 315, 319).

108. b An auditing process identifies risk areas such as chargemaster description, medical necessity, MS-DRG coding accuracy, variations in case mix, and the like. Admission diagnosis and complaints, clinical laboratory results, and radiology orders are not risk areas that should be targeted for audit (Schraffenberger and Kuehn 2011, 396–398).

109. a The compliance program addresses the coding function. Because the accuracy and completeness of ICD-10-CM and ICD-10-PCS for inpatient code assignment determine the provider payment, the coding compliance program should regularly audit these codes. It is important that healthcare organizations have a strong coding compliance program (Foltz and Lankisch 2020, 518–519; Schraffenberger and Palkie 2022, 4–5).

110. c Team members work together to assess and monitor denials. The team establishes goals and sets metrics and key performance indicators to support them. Three key goals of a denials management team are as follows: reduce the number of denials (lower denial rate); identify the source of denials; and develop physician and staff knowledge of documentation, coding, and billing regulations (Casto and White 2021, 220).

111. d The Comprehensive Error Rate Testing (CERT) program measures improper payments in various healthcare settings for Medicare (Casto and White 2021, 203).

112. b As part of this utilization review process, the case manager reviews for medical necessity and appropriateness. This utilization review process helps to improve patient outcomes and lower healthcare spending, while still providing appropriate care to patients at the appropriate time (Shaw and Carter 2019, 140).

113. b Clinical validation audits are conducted to determine if health records contain the necessary documentation, such as lab results, diagnostic test results, operative reports, and so forth to support the diagnoses made by the physician. Historically, physicians were able to diagnose conditions and diseases without supportive proof; however, those days are in the past. Providers who do not have health record documentation that substantiates their diagnoses will likely experience reductions in payment or denials of payment (Foltz and Lankisch 2020, 514–515).

114. b Physicians and other practitioners are notified when they have incomplete health records requiring their attention. If a health record remains incomplete for a specified number of days, as defined in the medical staff rules and regulations, the record is considered to be a delinquent record (Sayles 2020b, 77).

115. d Diversion is the removal of a medication from its usual stream of preparation, dispensing, and administration by personnel involved in those steps in order to use or sell the medication in nonhealthcare settings. An individual might take the medication for personal use, to sell on the street, to sell directly to a user as a dealer, or to sell to others who will redistribute for the diverting individual (Shaw and Carter 2019, 227–228).

116. c Over the past several years, the OIG has published several documents to help providers develop internal programs that include elements for ensuring compliance. One of the elements included is written policies and procedures (Foltz and Lankisch 2020, 511).

117. **a**   Implementation of an effective corporate compliance program significantly reduces the risk of unlawful or improper conduct, criminal or civil liability, and the risk of a government audit, and also promotes an ethical organizational culture (Bowman 2017, 437).

118. **b**   An example of unethical documentation in healthcare is retrospective documentation—when healthcare providers add documentation after care has been given, possibly for the purpose of increasing reimbursement or avoiding a medical legal action. The HIM professional is responsible for maintaining accurate and complete records and is able to identify the occurrence and either correct the error or indicate that the entry is a late entry into the health record (Hamilton 2020, 670–671).

119. **c**   Abuse occurs when a healthcare provider unknowingly or unintentionally submits an inaccurate claim for payment. Abuse generally results from unsound medical, business, or fiscal practices that directly or indirectly result in unnecessary costs to the Medicare program. The performance of medically unnecessary services and submitting them for payment would be an example of healthcare abuse (Casto and White 2021, 200).

120. **b**   Fraud in healthcare is defined as a deliberate false representation of fact, a failure to disclose a fact that is material (relevant) to a healthcare transaction, damage to another party that reasonably relies on the misrepresentation, or failure to disclose (Foltz and Lankisch 2020, 500).

121. **c**   The supervisor is responsible for ensuring turnaround times are met. Turnaround time is the time between receipt of the request and when the request is sent to the requester. The ROI system tracks requests for the information (Sayles 2020b, 69–70).

122. **a**   A corporate integrity agreement (CIA) is essentially a compliance program imposed by the government, with substantial government oversight and outside expert involvement in the organization's compliance activities. The OIG negotiates CIAs with healthcare providers and other entities as part of the settlement of federal healthcare program investigations arising under a variety of civil false claims statutes. Providers or entities agree to the obligations, and in exchange, OIG agrees not to seek their exclusion from participation in Medicare, Medicaid, or other federal healthcare programs (Bowman 2017, 460).

123. **d**   When a team examines a process with the intention of making improvements, it must first understand the process thoroughly. Each team member has a unique perspective and significant insight about how a portion of the process works. Flowcharts help all the team members understand the process in the same way (Carter and Palmer 2020, 563).

124. **a**   It is imperative that the RACs accurately identify improper payments. RACs must have a physician medical director as well as certified coding professionals on staff. For medical necessity reviews, many RACs use registered nurses or other clinical staff (Casto and White 2021, 205).

125. **c**   Physician practices use data analysis to ensure revenue integrity principles are being met. A big difference between facility E/M coding and physician practice E/M coding is that physicians are not able to use practice-specific criteria to assign E/M codes like facilities. Instead, they must follow strict E/M coding guidelines that are nationally recognized. Therefore, third-party payers often compare providers or group practices to each other to identify areas of variation. These areas of variation could be risk areas for the third-party payer. Payers perform audits to ensure that E/M coding is compliant with established coding guidelines. The concept of a bell-shaped curve for HCPCS codes that are natural levels may also be used when comparing the coding practices of physicians. Dr. Smith's bar graph shows a skew toward the higher level of visits, where the others do not. This could raise a red flag with a payer that the physician is inflating the actual visit work so an audit by the practice manager to assess the accuracy of the visit codes is warranted (Casto and White 2021, 236–237).

126. **a** A strong clinical documentation integrity (CDI) program is important to fighting fraud and abuse through the focus on quality and accuracy (Foltz and Lankisch 2020, 513).

127. **b** The data integrity analyst is responsible for ensuring the quality of the data in HIM information systems. Data integrity analysts must be able to apply data and content standards to data collection and data storage. They must be able to maintain the information systems, ensure compliance with legal and accreditation requirements, and analyze data (Sayles and Kavanaugh-Burke 2021,116).

128. **c** External audits are performed to confirm that a healthcare organization's internal audits are valid. In other words they help to ensure and validate that the internal audits identifying all of the compliance issues (Foltz and Lankisch 2020, 517).

129. **d** Benefits include improved documentation, high standard of coding, reduction in denials, and correction of coding-related risks (Foltz and Lankisch 2020, 518).

130. **b** Simple random sampling gives every bill, patient, and so forth the same chance of being chosen (Foltz and Lankisch 2020, 516).

131. **b** The author of the appeal letter should be appropriate for the type of the denial. For example, the physician would address medical necessity (Foltz and Lankisch 2020, 517).

132. **b** The CC capture rate is the number of patients with CCs compared to all of the patients in the population. With the changes in the CC list and the addition of MCCs in the MS-DRG system, facilities are finding that the CC capture rate is much lower than it had been previously, and new benchmarks need to be established for MS-DRGs. The CC capture rate is a valuable tool in measuring the overall severity of patients served by the facility as a whole or by a particular physician or specialty. Assuming that the coding is accurately completed, the rate can help measure the specificity of physician documentation (White 2021, 166).

133. **c** A hospital's case-mix index (CMI) represents the average MS-DRG relative weight for a particular hospital. The CMI allows administration to measure the hospital's performance based on MS-DRG cases. By analyzing a facility's CMI a manager is able to compare the CMI against other similar facilities in the area, or the year-to-year changes of the facility in its CMI. A decreasing CMI would indicate that the facility would be receiving decreased payment per case (Gordon, M. L. 2020, 493–494).

134. **c** The productivity increase with telecommuting is 20 percent. The facility has five coding professionals who are currently coding a total of 100 charts a day. With this 20 percent increase, each of the existing five coding professionals can code four records more per day each (a 20 percent increase). This amounts to 120 charts: 24 × 5 = 120. If the discharges increase by 44 charts, the facility would need one more FTE in the telecommuting staffing model, since each coding professional can code 24 records per day (White 2020, 157–158).

135. **d** Workload statistics can assist managers with the tasks of monitoring productivity and provide data regarding resources used, such as equipment, personnel, services, and supplies (Schraffenberger and Kuehn 2011, 223).

136. **d** Free-text data is the unstructured narrative data that is the result of a person typing data into an information system. It is undefined, unlimited, and unstructured, meaning that the typist can type anything into the field or document. The amount of free-text in the EHR should be limited as the ability to manipulate data is diminished with its use (Sayles 2020b, 82).

137. **c** It is not necessarily more difficult to manage remote staff; rather, it presents different challenges. In the remote environment, managers may need to rely on productivity and coding accuracy reports to determine the success of remote employees. When allowing coding professionals to work from home or contracting with remote coding professionals, work expectations must be established in advance (Prater 2020, 626–627).

138. **a** Most organizations create an electronic health records (EHR) steering committee to engage all the various stakeholders in EHR planning and development. This ensures that the EHR planning is comprehensive and also starts the process of introducing change and gaining buy-in (Amatayakul 2020, 351).

139. **c** Productivity standards should be based on both accuracy and volume (Prater 2020, 628–629)

140. **c** Work measurement is based on assessment of internal data collected on actual work performed within the organization and the calculation of time it takes to do the work (Prater 2020, 629).

141. **a** Collecting data on current performance and tasks allows the HIM supervisor to include all tasks that are being performed in the new job descriptions. When more than one person is performing a task, the data could be collected over time and averaged. One method of doing this is to keep a diary for a period of time on how they spend their time. The HIM supervisor may then use this data to revise the job description to accurately reflect the work performed (Prater 2020, 629–630).

142. **b** Reminders can notify physicians of screenings that should be performed based on the patient's age and gender. The other options are all alerts (Sayles 2020b, 83–84; Bowe and Williamson 2020, 370).

143. **a** It is generally agreed that Social Security numbers (SSNs) should not be used as patient identifiers. The Social Security Administration is adamant in its opposition to using the SSN for purposes other than those identified by law (Sayles 2020b, 84).

144. **a** In closure, the new system or process is used by the customer. This is the phase in which the project shifts to become an integrated part of organizational operations. During the operational phase, management must continually monitor performance and determine whether the new system or process meets established performance criteria (Shaw and Carter 2019, 371).

145. **c** Allowing employees of a covered entity to access their own protected health information electronically results in a situation in which the covered entity may be in compliance with parts of the HIPAA Privacy Rule but in violation of other sections of the Privacy Rule. An ideal situation would be to establish a patient portal through which all patients may view their own records in a secure manner and for which an employee has neither more or less rights than any other patient (Thomason 2013, 109).

146. **b** The HIPAA Privacy Rule allows individuals to decide whether they want to be listed in a facility directory when they are admitted to a facility. If the patient decides to be listed in the facility directory, the patient should be informed that only callers who know his or her name will be given any of this limited information. Covered entities generally do not, however, have to provide screening of visitors or calls for patients because such an activity is too difficult to manage with the number of employees and volunteers involved in the process of forwarding calls and directing visitors. If the covered entity agreed to the screening and could not meet the agreement, it could be considered a violation of this standard of the Privacy Rule (Thomason 2013, 105).

147. c   The education provided to the IT coordinator of the cardiology department was in regards to SNOWMED CT. The current version, Systematized Nomenclature of Medicine Clinical Terms (SNOMED CT), is the most comprehensive, multilingual clinical healthcare terminology in the world (Sayles and Kavanaugh-Burke 2021, 44).

148. a   Comparing an organization's performance to the performance of other organizations that provide the same types of service is known as benchmarking. Internal benchmarking is also important to establish a baseline for the organization to find ways to improve effectiveness (Shaw and Carter 2019, 42).

149. a   The monitoring activity is performed to determine the current status of the project, enabling the project to be controlled. The control activity is performed to assess project status in reference to planned activities and their timeline. If the project is off target, a project manager would take action to bring it back on track (Shaw and Carter 2019, 371).

150. a   One of two major ways to organize process work is serial work division, assembly line fashion, where tasks or steps are handled separately in sequence by multiple individuals (Prater 2020, 625).

Practice Question Answers

1. a   Healthcare data sets have two purposes. The first is to identify the data elements that should be collected for each patient. The second is to provide uniform definitions for common terms. The use of uniform definitions ensures that data collected from a variety of healthcare settings will share a standard definition. Standardizing data elements and definitions makes it possible to compare the data collected at different facilities (Brinda 2020, 156).

2. d   The purpose of the UHDDS is to list and define a set of common, uniform data elements. The data elements are collected from the health records of every hospital inpatient and later abstracted from the health record and included in national databases (Brinda 2020, 156).

3. d   A data dictionary is a listing of all the data elements within a specific information system that defines individual data element, standard input of the data element, and specific data length. A data dictionary should be implemented early by the organization to support standardization within the EHR (Brinda 2020, 155–156).

4. a   Analysis, or review, of the health record is performed by HIM department personnel to determine the completeness of the health record (Sayles 2020b, 76).

5. b   A data set is a list of recommended data elements with uniform definitions that are relevant for a particular use. The contents of data sets vary by their purpose. However, data sets are not meant to limit the number of data elements that can be collected. Most healthcare organizations collect additional data elements that have meaning for their specific administrative and clinical operations. Standardizing data elements and definitions makes it possible to compare the data collected at different facilities. A number of data reporting requirements come from federal initiatives (Brinda 2020, 156).

6. d   Technology has advanced to a point at which an unauthorized user can capture data in transit and alter it. Therefore, covered entities must confirm the integrity of data passed across a network. Integrity is the security principle that protects data from inappropriate modification or corruption. This includes both unintentional and intentional modifications and destructions. Unintentional modifications and destruction could occur if the wrong data are destroyed, the wrong backup is used to restore data, or an electrical fire destroys the computer (Sayles and Kavanaugh, 2021, 298–299).

7. a   A data set is a recommended list of data elements that have defined and uniformed definitions that are relevant for a particular use or are specific to a type of healthcare industry (Brinda 2020, 156).

8. a   Some providers also use a SOAP format for their problem-oriented progress notes. A subjective (S) entry relates significant information in the patient's words or from the patient's point of view (Huey 2021, 4).

9. b   Data granularity requires that the attributes and values of data be defined at the correct level of detail for the intended use of the data (Brinda 2020, 179–180).

10. c   Data are the raw elements that make up our communications. Humans have the innate ability to combine data they collect and, through all their senses, produce information (which is data that have been combined to produce value) and enhance that information with experience and trial-and-error that produces knowledge. In this example, the gender is tied to race in the data collection that constitutes information and not a data element (Fahrenholz 2017a, 72).

11. b   The continuity of care document (CCD) is a core data set of relevant administrative, demographic, and clinical information elements about a patient's health status and healthcare treatment. It was created to help communicate that information from one provider to another for referral, transfer, or discharge of the patient (Amatayakul 2020, 346).

12. b   The Outcomes and Assessment Information Set (OASIS) is a standardized data set designed to gather data about Medicare beneficiaries who are receiving services from a home health agency. OASIS includes a set of core data items that are collected on all adult home health patients (Selman-Holman 2017, 362).

13. a   Some providers also use a SOAP format for their problem-oriented progress notes. Professional conclusions reached from evaluation of the subjective or objective information make up the assessment (A) (Huey 2021, 4).

14. d   The ability to copy previous entries and paste into a current entry leads to a record in which a clinician may, upon signing the documentation, unwittingly swear to the accuracy and comprehensiveness of substantial amounts of duplicated or inapplicable information as well as the incorporation of misleading or erroneous documentation. The HIM professional plays a critical role in developing policies and procedures to ensure the integrity of patient information (Sayles 2020b, 82).

15. d   The Healthcare Effectiveness Data and Information Set (HEDIS) is sponsored by the National Committee for Quality Assurance (NCQA). HEDIS is a set of standard performance measures designed to provide healthcare purchasers and consumers with the information they need to compare the performance of healthcare plans (Shaw and Carter 2019, 332).

16. **b** Data consistency means that the data are reliable. Reliable data do not change no matter how many times or in how many ways they are stored, processed, or displayed. Data values are consistent when the value of any given data element is the same across applications and systems. Related data items also should be reliable (Brickner 2020b, 304).

17. **c** The operative report describes the surgical procedures performed on the patient. The operative report should be written or dictated by the surgeon immediately after surgery and become part of the health record (Brickner 2020a, 108–109).

18. **a** Data and content standards are clear guidelines for the acceptable values for specified data fields. These standards make it possible to exchange health information using electronic networks (Sayles and Kavanaugh-Burke 2021, 367).

19. **c** The data collected by the Minimum Data Set (MDS) are used to develop care plans for residents and to document placement at the appropriate level of care. The MDS provides a structured way to organize resident information and develop a resident care plan (Brickner 2020a, 112).

20. **a** Patient care delivery is a primary purpose of the health record. Other primary purposes are patient care management, patient care support processes, financial and other administrative processes, and patient self-management (Sayles 2020b, 64).

21. **b** Data accessibility means that the data are obtainable. Any organization that maintains health records for individual patients must have systems in place that identify each patient and support efficient access to information on each patient. Authorized users of the health record must be able to access information easily when and where they need it (Brinda 2020, 179).

22. **a** The EHR improves the quality of care because of the immediate access to patient information, as well as the use of alerts and reminders built into the system. These types of alerts help prevent medication errors, facilitate the notification of abnormal test results, and improve the quality of care through validation mechanisms (Sayles and Kavanaugh-Burke 2021, 63).

23. **a** The results of all diagnostic and therapeutic procedures become part of the patient's health record. The laboratory report includes tests performed on blood, urine, and other samples from the patient (Brickner 2020a, 108).

24. **b** The discharge summary is a concise account of the patient's illness, course of treatment, response to treatment, and condition at the time the patient is discharged (officially released) from the hospital. The summary also includes instructions for follow-up care to be given to the patient or his or her caregiver at the time of discharge. It provides an overview of the entire health encounter. The discharge summary is the responsibility of, and must be signed by, the attending physician (Brickner 2020a, 109).

25. **c** Data granularity requires that the attributes and values of data be defined at the correct level of detail for the intended use of the data. For example, numerical values for laboratory results should be recorded to the appropriate decimal place as required for the meaningful interpretation of test results—or in the collection of demographic data, data elements should be defined appropriately to determine the differences in outcomes of care among various populations (Brinda 2020, 179–180).

26. **a** The health record generally contains two types of data—clinical and administrative. Clinical data document the patient's health condition, diagnosis, and procedures performed as well as the healthcare treatment provided. Administrative data include demographic and financial information as well as various consents and authorizations related to the provision of care and the handling of confidential patient information (Brickner 2020a, 104).

27. **c** Data currency and data timeliness mean that healthcare data should be up-to-date and recorded at or near the time of the event or observation. Because care and treatment rely on accurate and current data, an essential characteristic of data quality is the timeliness of the documentation or data entry (Brinda 2020, 179).

28. **b** The health record number is a key data element in the master patient index (MPI). It is used as a unique personal identifier and is also used in paper-based numerical filing systems to locate records and in electronic systems to link records. Although it is typically assigned at the point of patient registration, the HIM department is usually responsible for the integrity of health record number assignment and for ensuring that no two patients receive the same number (Sayles 2020b, 70–71).

29. **d** This documentation would typically be found in social service notes (Fahrenholz 2013c, 402).

30. **d** When a deficiency is identified in the health record, it must be corrected. This may require locating a missing document or asking the physician or other healthcare provider to either sign or complete a document (Sayles 2020b, 76–77).

31. **a** A patient portal is specific software that enables patients to log on to a website from home or a kiosk in a provider's waiting room to have access some of their health information and other services including the ability to upload information for review by their provider (Amatayakul 2020, 346).

32. **b** A complete medical history documents the patient's current complaints and symptoms and lists his or her past health, personal, and family history. In acute care, the health history is usually the responsibility of the attending physician (Brickner 2020a, 104).

33. **a** Nurses maintain chronological records of the patient's vital signs (blood pressure, heart rate, respiration rate, and temperature) and separate logs that show what medications were ordered and when they were administered on the medication administration record (MAR) (Hunt 2017, 188).

34. **b** The consultation report documents the clinical opinion of a physician other than the primary or attending physician. The consultation is requested by the primary or attending physician. The report is based on the consulting physician's examination of the patient and a review of his or her health record (Brickner 2020a, 109).

35. **c** The secondary purposes of the health record are not associated with specific encounters between patient and healthcare professional. Rather, they are related to the environment in which patient care is provided. Some secondary purposes are support for research, to serve as evidence in litigation, to allocate resources, to plan market strategy, and the like (Sayles 2020b, 65).

36. **d** Information usually documented in the physical examination includes vital signs and examinations of the head, eyes, ears, nose, throat (HEENT) (Brickner 2020a, 104–106).

37. c Backscanning is the process of scanning past health records into the document management system (DMS) so there is an existing database of patient information, making the DMS valuable to the user from the first day of implementation (Sayles and Kavanugh-Burke 2021, 177).

38. a The barcode makes indexing more efficient because the barcode can enter metadata automatically. Standards for the use of barcodes must be established to facilitate scanning. These standards should include the size of the barcode, the standardized location of the barcode, and the amount of white space between the barcode and any text (Sayles and Kavanugh-Burke 2021, 178).

39. c Reliability refers to the degree to which a selection test produces consistent scores on a test and retest. Reliability is frequently checked by having more than one person abstract data for the same case. The results are then compared to identify any discrepancies (Prater 2020, 622–623).

40. a The consultation report documents the clinical opinion of a physician other than the primary or attending physician. The consultation is requested by the primary or attending physician. The report is based on the consulting physician's examination of the patient and a review of his or her health record (Brickner 2020a, 109).

41. a The physical examination report represents the attending physician's assessment of the patient's current health status. This report should document data on all the patient's major organ systems (Brickner 2020a, 104–106).

42. c Data comprehensiveness means that all the required data elements are included in the health record. In essence, comprehensiveness means that the record is complete. In both paper-based and computer-based systems, having a complete health record is critical to the organization's ability to provide excellent patient care and to meet all regulatory, legal, and reimbursement requirements (Brinda 2020, 179).

43. b The law requires healthcare facilities to query the National Practitioner Data Bank (NPDB) as part of the credentialing process. The database should be queried when a physician initially applies for medical staff privileges and every two years thereafter (Sharp 2020, 211–212).

44. d Policies and procedures need to be in place to address amendments and corrections in the EHR. Once a document is authenticated, the document should be locked to prevent changes. In the event that an amendment, addendum, or deletion needs to be made, the document would need to be unlocked. The EHR should retain the previous version of the document and identify who made the change along with the date and time that the change was made (Sayles 2020b, 83).

45. d Patients are individual users of the health record. Patients are informed consumers of their healthcare. As informed consumers, patients may obtain access to and be informed about their health record through copies of records or via a personal health record (Sayles 2020b, 66).

46. b A review of the identified duplicates and overlays often reveals procedural problems that contribute to the creation of errors. Although health information management (HIM) departments may be the hub of identifying, mitigating, and correcting master patient index (MPI) errors, that information may never be shared with the registration department. If the registration staff is not aware of the errors, how can they begin to proactively prevent the errors from occurring in the first place? Registration process improvement activities can eventually reduce work for HIM departments (Sayles 2020b, 72).

47. c   The copy and paste functionality in the electronic health record can result in incorrect information being copied into the health record (Sayles 2020b, 82).

48. b   The quality of the documentation entered in the health record by providers can have major impacts on the ability of coding staff to perform their clinical analyses and assign accurate codes. In this situation, the best solution would be to educate the entire medical staff on their roles in the clinical documentation improvement process. Explaining to them the documentation guidelines and what documentation is needed in the record to support the more accurate coding of diabetes and its manifestations will reduce the need for coding professionals to continue to query for this clarification (Foltz and Lankisch 2020, 521–522).

49. b   Validity is the degree to which codes accurately reflect the patient's diagnoses and procedures (Prater 2020, 622).

50. c   The Outcomes and Assessment Information Set (OASIS) consists of data elements that represent core items for the comprehensive assessment of an adult home care patient and form the basis for measuring patient outcomes for the purpose of outcome-based quality improvement (Selman-Holman 2017, 362).

51. a   Accreditation is the act of granting approval to a healthcare organization. The approval is based on whether the organization has met a set of voluntary standards that were developed by the accreditation agency. Voluntary reviews are conducted at the request of the healthcare facility seeking accreditation or certification. The Joint Commission is an example of an accreditation agency (Shaw and Carter 2019, 330).

52. d   The Joint Commission has been the most visible organization responsible for accrediting healthcare organizations since the mid-1950s. The primary focus of the Joint Commission at this time is to determine whether organizations seeking accreditation are continually monitoring the quality of the care they provide. The Joint Commission requires that this continual improvement process be in place throughout the entire organization, from the governing body down, as well as across all department lines (Shaw and Carter 2019, 330).

53. a   Every healthcare organization should have a clinical forms or design (for EHR systems) committee. This committee should provide oversight for the development, review, and control of all enterprise-wide information capture tools, including paper forms and design of computer screens (Sayles 2020b, 79).

54. d   It is important the informed consent be completed to ensure that the patient has a basic understanding of diagnosis and the nature of the treatment or procedure, along with the risks, benefits, alternatives (including opting out of treatment), and individuals who will perform the treatment or procedure. Information consent is a process and it is the responsibility of the provider or physician who will be rendering the treatment or performing the procedure to obtain the patient's informed consent and answer the patient's questions (Rinehart-Thompson 2020a, 231).

55. c   A care plan is a summary of the patient's problems from the nurse or other professional's perspective with a detailed plan for interventions that may follow the assessment (Brickner 2020a, 107).

56. **b** An on-site review by experienced surveyor from the accrediting organization would meet with the HIM leader to review their written policies and procedures and ask for some examples of the HIM department's successes in areas of quality improvement and patient safety. The type of successes the surveyor would be looking for might be that the signing, dating, and timing of physician verbal orders went from 95 percent compliance to 99 percent. Another success would be the reduction of duplicate or overlaid medical record numbers (MRN) (Rossiter 2017, 290).

57. **a** The Commission on Accreditation of Rehabilitation Facilities (CARF) is a private, not-for-profit organization committed to developing and maintaining practical, customer-focused standards to help organizations measure and improve the quality, value, and outcomes of behavioral health and medical rehabilitation programs. CARF accreditation is based on an organization's commitment to continually enhance the quality of its services and programs and to focus on customer satisfaction (Shaw and Carter 2019, 331).

58. **a** The data dictionary is a central building block that supports communication across business processes. Defining a data dictionary supports the creation of well-structured and defined data sets by creating standardized definitions of data elements to help ensure consistency of collection and use of the data. For example, the data element "PATIENT" would have the same field length and definition across all applications in the organization (Brinda 2020, 155–156).

59. **d** The Joint Commission requires healthcare organizations to conduct in-depth investigations of occurrences that resulted—or could have resulted—in life-threatening injuries to patients, medical staff, visitors, and employees. The Joint Commission uses the term *sentinel event* for such occurrences (Carter and Palmer 2020, 553).

60. **b** Interoperability refers to the use of standard protocols to enable two different computer systems to share data with each other (Brinda 2020, 174).

61. **c** Because the United States does not have a national patient identifier, an identity matching algorithm process must be used by organizations to identify any patient for whom data are to be exchanged. This algorithm uses sophisticated probability equations to identify patients (Amatayakul 2020, 348).

62. **c** Good forms design is needed within an EHR to create ease of use. The use of a selection box allows the user to select a value from a predefined list. Check boxes are used for multiple selections and radio buttons are used for single selections (Sayles 2020b, 83–84).

63. **a** The vocabulary used in an electronic health record (EHR) system should, at a minimum, be a controlled vocabulary, which is essential in ensuring a common meaning for all users. A controlled vocabulary means that a specific set of terms in the EHR's data dictionary may be used and that a central authority approves any additions or changes (Amatayakul 2017, 290).

64. **d** Point of care documentation informs the user (clinician) what data needs to be recorded for the patient and to use that data to supply clinical decision support, including alerts and reminders, at the time when the clinician is able to be most responsive to alerts and reminders, therefore ensuring timely documentation (Amatayakul, 2020, 334).

65. **b** Data is collected in a number of ways. The information system should have measures in place to control the data entered into the EHR. In this example, the birth date of 10101963 is displayed in the computer as 10/10/1963 because an input mask was used in the information system to show the format in which the data will be displayed (Sayles 2020b, 83).

66. **a** An information silo is where information is not shared within a department that does not integrate into the main organizational system nor can others access it outside of that specific department (Amatayakul 2017, 223)

67. **a** Within each chapter, the standards associated with each topic are cited and then elaborated upon with "elements of performance" (EP) that directly communicate the intent of the Joint Commission with respect to each standard. In addition, a scoring guideline is provided that allows the organization to score itself on each EP and thus get a sum total on each standard (Shaw and Carter 2019, 331).

68. **d** Data comprehensiveness means that all the required data elements are included in the health record. In essence, comprehensiveness means that the record is complete. In both paper-based and computer-based systems, having a complete health record is critical to the organization's ability to provide excellent patient care and to meet all regulatory, legal, and reimbursement requirements (Brinda 2020, 179).

69. **c** Quantitative analysis is used by health information management professionals as a method to detect whether elements of the patient's health record are missing, or not complete (Sayles and Kavanaugh-Burke 2021, 23–24).

70. **a** Healthcare Effectiveness Data and Information Set (HEDIS) is overseen by the National Committee for Quality Assurance. HEDIS is a standardized set of performance measures designed to allow purchasers to compare the performance of managed-care plans (Shaw and Carter 2019, 332).

71. **b** Qualitative analysis is a detailed review of a patient's health record for the quality of the documentation contained therein (Sayles and Kavanaugh-Burke 2021, 24).

72. **a** Create a matrix that defines each document type in the legal health record and determine the medium in which each element will appear. Such a matrix could include a column indicating the transition date of a particular document from the paper-based to the electronic environment. It is important that specific state guidelines are incorporated when a facility matrix is developed (Fahrenholz 2017c, 53).

73. **a** Even if evidence appears to be relevant, it must also be authenticated. As with health records, the evidence itself must be shown to have a baseline authenticity or trustworthiness (Klaver 2017a, 78).

74. **a** The data element PATIENT_LAST_NAME should be stored as alphanumeric data because the data are character-based (Brinda 2020, 155–156).

75. **b** General documentation guidelines apply to all categories of health records (Brickner 2020a, 101).

76. **a** Behavioral health records are more commonly referred to as mental health records and contain much of the same content as a nonbehavioral health record such as discharge summary, H&P, or physician's orders. Behavioral health records contain a treatment plan that often includes family and caregiver input and information as well as assessments geared toward the transition to outpatient, nonacute treatment (Brickner 2020a, 113).

77. **a** In the EHR, the user is able to copy and paste free text from one patient or patient encounter to another. This practice is dangerous as inaccurate information can easily be copied and information can be outdated (Sayles 2020b, 82).

78. b   The long-term care health record contains the patient's registration forms, personal property list, RAI and MDS, care plan, and discharge or transfer information (Brickner 2020a, 111–112).

79. b   Data stewardship is the evaluation of the data collection based on business need and strategy to ensure the data meets the requirements of patient care and organizational needs. Data stewardship and data ownership are closely connected (Brinda 2020, 171–172).

80. a   A data element can be a single or individual fact that represents the smallest unique subset of a larger database, sometimes referred to as the raw facts and figures (Brinda 2020, 155).

81. c   The Joint Commission uses tracer methodology for on-site surveys. The tracer methodology follows the experience of care through the organization's entire healthcare process, and allows the surveyor to identify performance issues (Rinehart-Thompson 2017e, 263).

82. c   Quantitative analysis is used by health information management technicians as a method to detect whether elements of the patient's health record are missing (Sayles and Kavanaugh-Burke 2021, 23–24).

83. b   When a case is first entered in the registry, an accession number is assigned. This number consists of the first digits of the year the patient was first seen at the facility, and the remaining digits are assigned sequentially throughout the year. The first case in the year, for example, might be 10-0001. The accession number may be assigned manually or by the automated cancer database used by the organization (Sharp 2020, 203).

84. d   Data also are categorized as either patient identifiable data, or aggregate data. With patient identifiable data, the patient is identified within the data either by name or number. The health record consists entirely of patient-identified data (Sharp 2020, 198).

85. c   Trauma registries maintain databases on patients with severe traumatic injuries. A traumatic injury is a wound or other injury caused by an external physical force such as an automobile accident, a shooting, a stabbing, or a fall (Sharp 2020, 204–205).

86. d   Promoting interoperability (formally referred to as meaningful use) is criteria with specific objectives and measures to be met by hospitals to demonstrate they are using EHRs that positively affect patient care (Johns 2015, 33–34).

87. c   The master patient index assigns a unique patient identifier to a patient. This facilitates managing a patient's multiple encounters as a "unit" over the course of a lifetime (Johns 2015, 55).

88. d   Embedded metadata are most often associated with automated records of operations (such as audit trails) and are stored with the date themselves. If data move from a source system to another system, then the system can attach metadata that identify where the data originated. In this way, metadata helps track data movement from one system to another (Johns 2015, 145).

89. a   A constraint is a condition that determines what values an attribute or relationship can or must have, which is one of the business rule categories (Johns 2015, 153).

90. b   In a forward map, an older version of a code set is mapped to a newer version (Johns 2015, 285).

91. d   Data integrity means that data are complete, accurate, consistent, and up-to-date so it is reliable (Brickner 2020b, 286).

92. c   Information governance is the accountability framework and decision rights to achieve enterprise information management. In other words, the information must be controlled to ensure the needs of the organization are met (Sayles 2020a, 6–7).

93. c   Data comprehensiveness means that all the required data elements are included in the health record. In essence, comprehensiveness means that the record is complete. In both paper-based and computer-based systems, having a complete health record is critical to the organization's ability to provide excellent patient care and to meet all regulatory, legal, and reimbursement requirements (Brinda 2020, 179).

94. b   General documentation guidelines apply to all categories of health records. Every healthcare organization should have policies that ensure the uniformity of both the content and format of the health record. These policies should be based on all applicable accreditation standards (Brickner 2020a, 101).

95. a   The primary purposes of the health record are related to providing care to the patient. Patient care includes the direct care provided and the day-to-day business of the organization (Sayles 2020b, 64–65).

96. d   The Joint Commission accredits rehabilitation programs and services but they do not focus on it like CARF does (Brickner 2020a, 98, 113).

97. a   Hospitals accredited through the Joint Commission or another accrediting body may participate in the Medicare program because the accrediting agency has been granted deemed status by the Medicare program. Deemed status means accrediting bodies such as the Joint Commission can survey facilities for compliance with the Medicare Conditions of Participation for Hospitals instead of the government (Rinehart-Thompson 2017e, 253).

98. d   Knowledge consists of a combination of rules, relationships, ideas, and experiences applied to information. The statement "Mary Jones's hemoglobin of 13 is within normal range" identifies the patient, specific information about that patient, and how it relates to normal parameters, which makes it knowledge rather than information (Johns 2015, 25).

99. b   The results of all diagnostic and therapeutic procedures become part of the patient's health record. Diagnostic procedures include laboratory tests performed on blood, urine, and other samples from the patient that would be documented in the laboratory findings (Brickner 2020a, 108).

100. b   Clinical documentation best practices establish policies and guidelines that ensure uniformity of both content and format of the patient record. One example of a clinical documentation best practice would be to stipulate abbreviations and symbols in the patient record to be permitted only when approved according to hospital and medical staff bylaws, rules, and regulations (Johns 2015, 13).

101. c   Dr. Hall must document a new history and physical for Mary because the last history and physical was completed 60 days ago. A history and physical must be completed within 30 days of admission or within 24 hours after admission. If a history and physical is completed within 30 days of a surgery, an updated exam must be documented within 24 hours of admission and prior to the surgery or procedure (Brickner 2020a, 97).

102. **d**　The following list identifies some of the most common components of long-term care records: registration forms including resident identification data, personal property list, history and physical and hospital records, advance directives, bill of rights, and other legal records, and RAI and care plan (Brickner 2020a, 111–112).

103. **c**　This is an example of a patient portal sending messages (email alert and notification) directly to a patient on needed healthcare visit (Amayatakul 2020, 346).

104. **d**　There are important applications that support electronic health record (EHR) functionality. Many hospitals begin their EHR implementation with point-of-care (POC) charting systems. These might include nursing admission assessments, nursing progress notes, vital signs charting, intake and output records, and the like (Bowe and Williamson, 2020, 367–368).

105. **d**　Data governance is the enterprise authority that ensures control and accountability for enterprise data through the establishment of decision rights and data policies and standards that are implemented and monitored through a formal structure of assigning roles, responsibilities, and accountabilities. Promoting the sale of data would not be a role of data governance (Johns 2015, 81).

106. **b**　A reverse map links two systems in the opposite direction, from the newer version of a code set to an older version (Johns 2015, 285).

107. **c**　Structured data entry techniques constrain data capture into a common format or vocabulary. A purpose of structured data entry is to reduce variability in terminology, allowing for standardization (Johns 2015, 231).

108. **b**　Data elements in a deterministic algorithm are used to disqualify two or more similar records, rather than match them. These should be static attributes that do not normally change such as date of birth (Sayles 2020b, 72).

109. **c**　An overlap is when one entity has different unique identifiers in different databases (Johns 2015, 177).

110. **a**　One example of effective form design principles is that each form should include original and revised dates for the tracking and purging of obsolete forms (Sayles 2020b, 78).

111. **c**　Data security includes ensuring that workstations are protected from unauthorized access. If a workstation is inactive for a period of time specified by the organization, it should log itself off automatically. The automatic log-off helps prevent unauthorized users from accessing e-PHI when an authorized user walks away from the computer without logging out of the system (Sayles and Kavanaugh-Burke 2021, 297).

112. **d**　Security awareness requires entities to provide security training for all staff. They must address security reminders, detection and reporting of malicious software, log-in monitoring, and password management. Edit checks, audit trails, and password management can all be programmed to be automatic controls where a security awareness program cannot (Brickner 2020b, 308).

113. **a**　The security audit process should include triggers that identify the need for a closer inspection. These trigger events cannot be used as the sole basis of the review, but they can significantly reduce the amount of reviews performed. An example of a trigger is when a user has the same last name as patient (Sayles and Kavanaugh-Burke 2021, 298).

114. **a** The master patient index (MPI) is the permanent record of all patients treated at a healthcare facility. It is used by the HIM department to look up patient demographics, dates of care, the patient's health record number, and other information (Sayles 2020b, 70–71).

115. **a** An audit trail is a software program that tracks every single access or attempted access of data in the computer system. It logs the name of the individual who accessed the data, terminal location or IP address, the date and time accessed, the type of data, and the action taken (for example, modifying, reading, or deleting data) (Brickner 2020b, 301).

116. **a** A contingency plan is a standard that requires the establishment and implementation of policies and procedures for responding to emergencies or failures in systems that contain e-PHI. It includes a data backup plan, disaster recovery plan, emergency mode of operation plan, testing and revision procedures, and applications and data criticality analysis to prioritize data and determine what must be maintained or restored first in an emergency (Brickner 2020b, 308).

117. **b** HIPAA allows the covered entity to impose a reasonable cost-based fee when the individual requests a copy of PHI or agrees to accept summary or explanatory information. The fee may include the cost of copying, including supplies, labor, and postage. HIPAA does not permit retrieval fees to be charged to patients (Rinehart-Thompson 2020b, 255).

118. **d** Section 164.524 of the Privacy Rule states that an individual has a right of access to inspect and obtain a copy of his or her own protected health information (PHI) that is contained in a designated record set, such as a health record. The individual's right extends for as long as the PHI is maintained. However, there are exceptions to what PHI may be accessed. For example, psychotherapy notes; information compiled in reasonable anticipation of a civil, criminal, or administrative action or proceeding; or PHI subject to the Clinical Laboratory Improvements Act (CLIA) are all exceptions (Rinehart-Thompson 2020b, 254).

119. **c** The HIPAA Privacy Rule provides patients with significant rights that allow them to have some measure of control over their health information. As long as state laws or regulations or the physician does not state otherwise (such as when a licensed healthcare professional has determined that access would likely endanger the life or safety of the individual) competent adult patients have the right to access their health record (Rinehart-Thompson 2017d, 243–244).

120. **a** Within the context of data security, protecting data privacy means safeguarding access to information. Only those individuals who need to know information should be authorized to access it (Johns 2015, 210–211).

121. **b** All data security policies and procedures should be reviewed and evaluated annually to make sure they are up-to-date and still relevant to the organization (Brickner 2020b, 306).

122. **a** Risk management begins by conducting a risk analysis. Identifying security threats or risks, determining how likely it is that any given threat may occur, and estimating the impact of an untoward event are all parts of a risk assessment (Brickner 2020b, 296).

123. **d** Access to e-PHI can be controlled through the use of the following: user-based access, role-based access, and context-based access. Role-based access control decisions are based on the roles individual users have as part of an organization. Each user is given various privileges to perform their role or function (Brickner 2020b, 297).

124. b   Administrative safeguards include policies and procedures that address the management of computer resources. For example, one such policy might direct users to log off the computer system when they are not using it or employ automatic log-offs after a period of inactivity (Brickner 2020b, 300).

125. c   Employees are the biggest threat to the security of healthcare data. Whether it is disgruntled employees destroying computer hardware, snooping employees accessing information without authorization, or employees accessing information for fraudulent purposes, employees are a real threat to data security (Brickner 2020b, 288–289).

126. b   Data security can be defined as the protection measures and tools for safeguarding information and information systems (Brickner 2020b, 286).

127. c   The HIM supervisor should determine if a breach has occurred before action is taken. This can be done using an audit trail, which is a software program that tracks access to data in the EHR. It logs the name of the individual who accessed the data, the date and time, and the action taken (for example, modifying, reading, or deleting data) (Brickner 2020b, 301).

128. c   Physical safeguards protect physical equipment, media, or facilities. For example, doors leading to the areas that house mainframes and other principal computing equipment should have locks on them (Brickner 2020b, 299–300).

129. a   Review of records by the patient is permitted after the authorization for use and disclosure is verified. Usually hospital personnel should be present during on-site reviews to assist the requester with the paper record or working with the EHR if necessary. Assistance would not be needed if the people requesting on-site review work for the facility (Rinehart-Thompson 2020b, 254–255).

130. c   The HIPAA Privacy Rule provides patients with significant rights that allow them to have some measure of control over their health information. As long as state laws or regulations or the physician do not state otherwise, competent adult patients have the right to access their health record (Rinehart-Thompson 2017d, 243–244).

131. c   Single sign-on allows sign-on to multiple related, but independent, software systems. With this property a user logs in once and gains access to all systems without being prompted to log in again at each of them. Single sign-off is the reverse property whereby a single action of signing out terminates access to multiple software systems (Brickner 2020b, 299).

132. b   Physical safeguards protect physical equipment, media, or facilities. For example, doors leading to the areas that house mainframes and other principal computing equipment should have locks on them Brickner 2020b, 299–300).

133. b   The term *access control* means being able to identify which employees should have access to what data. The general practice is that employees should have access only to data they need to do their jobs. For example, an admitting clerk and a healthcare provider would not have access to the same kinds of data (Brickner 2020b, 297–298).

134. c   Because HIPAA defers to state laws on the issue of minors, applicable state laws should be consulted regarding appropriate authorization. In general, the age of maturity is 18 years or older. This is the legal recognition that an individual is considered responsible for, and has control over, his or her actions (Klaver 2017b, 160).

135. c   A secure patient-provider portal allows for the communication between the provider and the patient and is not just a site for patients to access information. This is part of the effort to engage patients in their care (Sayles and Kavanaugh-Burke 2021, 209).

136. b   User-based access is a security mechanism that grants users of a system access based on their identity (Brickner 2020b, 297).

137. d   A portal is a special application to provide secure remote access to specific applications (Amatayakul 2017, 15).

138. a   Since this breach applies to one patient, it must be reported to HHS within 60 days after the end of the calendar year (Rinehart-Thompson 2020b, 271).

139. c   Strong authentication requires providing information from two of the three different types of authentication information. The three methods are something you know such as a password or PIN; something you have, such as an ATM card, token, swipe card, or smart card; and something you are, such as a biometric fingerprint, voice scan, iris, or retinal scan. An individual who provides something he knows (password) and something he has (swipe card) is called two-factor authentication (Brickner 2020b, 298–299).

140. b   A healthcare organization must be able to replace data if a server or storage device is destroyed in some manner, but organizations need to be able to instantaneously failover to another server during a server crash. Back up of stored data has been routinely performed by most healthcare organizations. To reduce the risk of downtime, healthcare organizations now must also have server redundancy with server failover (Sayles and Kavanaugh-Burke 2021, 292).

141. a   In order for an authorization to be valid, it must contain an expiration date or event that relates to the individual or the purpose of the use or disclosure (Rinehart-Thompson 2020b, 276).

142. c   One security strategy is to implement application safeguards. These are controls contained in the application software or computer programs. One common application control is password management. It involves keeping a record of end users' identifications and passwords and then matching the passwords to each end user's privileges (Brickner 2020b, 301).

143. a   Metadata are data about data and include information that track actions such as when and by whom a document was accessed or changed, such as in an audit log (Rinehart-Thompson 2020a, 228).

144. d   Determining what data to make available to an employee usually involves identifying classes of information based on the employee's role in the organization. Every role in the organization should be identified, along with the type of information required to perform it. This is often referred to as role-based access. Although there are other types of access control strategies, role-based access is probably the one used most often in healthcare organizations. Access to information and information resources (such as computers) must be restricted to those authorized to access the information or the associated resources (Brickner 2020b, 297–298).

145. b   Disaster planning occurs through a contingency plan—a set of procedures documented by the organization to be followed when responding to emergencies. It encompasses what an organization and its personnel need to do both during and after events that limit or prevent access to facilities and patient information (Brickner 2020b, 303–304).

146. **d** An outsourced transcription company and vendor would be business associates of a covered entity (CE). Although business associates are not directly regulated by the Privacy Rule, they do come under the Privacy Rule's requirements by virtue of their association with one or more CEs. A business associate is a person or organization other than a member of a CE's workforce that performs functions or activities on behalf of or affecting a CE that involve the use or disclosure of individually identifiable health information (45 CFR 160.103(1); Rinehart-Thompson 2017c, 210–211).

147. **d** With the passage of the Privacy Rule, a minimum amount of protection (that is, a floor) was achieved uniformly across all the states through the establishment of a consistent set of standards that affected providers, healthcare clearinghouses, and health plans (Rinehart-Thompson 2017c, 210).

148. **c** To meet the individually identifiable element of PHI, the information must meet all three portions of a three-part test: it must either identify the person or provide a reasonable basis to believe the person could be identified from the information given; it must relate to one's past, present, or future physical or mental health condition, the provision of healthcare, or payment for the provision of healthcare; and it must be held or transmitted by a covered entity or its business associate (Rinehart-Thompson 2017c, 213).

149. **b** The audit trail is a software program that tracks every single access to data in the computer system. It logs the name of the individual who accessed the data, the date and time, and the action taken (for example, modifying, reading, or deleting data). Review of audit trails can help detect whether a breach of security has occurred (Brickner 2020b, 301).

150. **c** There are certain circumstances where the minimum necessary requirement does not apply, such as to healthcare providers for treatment; to the individual or his personal representative; pursuant to the individual's authorization to the secretary of the HHS for investigations, compliance review, or enforcement; as required by law; or to meet other Privacy Rule compliance requirements (Rinehart-Thompson 2017c, 232–233).

151. **d** Covered entities (CEs) are responsible for their workforce, which consists not only of employees but also volunteers, student interns, and trainees. Workforce members are not limited to those who receive wages from the CE (45 CFR 160.103; Rinehart-Thompson 2017c, 210–211).

152. **d** Vendors who have a presence in a healthcare facility, agency, or organization will often have access to patient information in the course of their work. If the vendor meets the definition of a business associate (that is, it is using or disclosing an individual's PHI on behalf of the healthcare organization), a business associate agreement must be signed. If a vendor is not a business associate, employees of the vendor should sign confidentiality agreements because of their routine contact with and exposure to patient information. In this situation, Ready-Clean is not a business associate (Brodnik 2017b, 211).

153. **c** Implementation specifications define how standards are to be implemented. Implementation specifications are either "required" or "addressable." Covered entities must implement all implementation specifications that are required. For those implementation specifications that are labeled addressable, the covered entity must conduct a risk assessment and evaluate whether the specification is appropriate to its environment (Brickner 2020b, 307).

154. **d** Competent adults have a general right to consent to or refuse medical treatment. In general, a competent adult has the right to request, receive, examine, copy, and authorize disclosure of the patient's healthcare information (Brodnik 2017b, 341).

155. **c** Administrative safeguards are documented, formal practices to manage data security measures throughout the organization. Basically, they require the facility to establish a security management process. The administrative provisions detail how the security program should be managed from the organization's perspective. Administrative safeguards have nine standards, including the development and testing of a contingency plan. This is to ensure that procedures are in place to handle an emergency response in the event of an untoward event such as a power outage (Brickner 2020b, 308).

156. **d** The Business Records Exception is the rule under which a record is determined not to be hearsay if it was made at or near the time by, or from information transmitted by, a person with knowledge; it was kept in the course of a regularly conducted business activity; and it was the regular practice of that business activity to make the record (Klaver 2017a, 80).

157. **b** Although a person or organization may, by definition, be subject to the Privacy Rule by virtue of the type of organization it is, not all information that it holds or comes into contact with is protected by the Privacy Rule. For example, the Privacy Rule has specifically excluded from its scope employment records held by the covered entity in its role as employer (45 CFR 160.103). Under this exclusion, employee physical examination reports contained within personnel files are specifically exempted from this rule (Rinehart-Thompson 2017c, 215).

158. **b** Because of cost and space limitations, permanently storing paper and microfilm-based health record documents is not an option for most hospitals. Acceptable destruction methods for paper documents include burning, shredding, pulping, and pulverizing (Fahrenholz 2017a, 107).

159. **a** The Privacy Rule introduced the standard of minimum necessary to limit the amount of PHI used, disclosed, and requested. This means that healthcare providers and other covered entities must limit uses, disclosures, and requests to only the amount needed to accomplish the intended purpose. For example, for payment purposes, only the minimum amount of information necessary to substantiate a claim for payment should be disclosed (Rinehart-Thompson 2020b, 253).

160. **b** The Privacy Rule introduced the standard that individuals should be informed how covered entities use or disclose protected health information (PHI). Section 164.520 requires that, except for certain variations or exceptions for health plans and correctional facilities, an individual has the right to a notice explaining how his or her PHI will be used and disclosed. This is the notice of privacy practices (Rinehart-Thompson 2020b, 260–262).

161. **b** Agreements between the covered entity and a business associate include requiring the business associate to make available all of its books and records relating to protected health information (PHI) use and disclosure to the Department of Health and Human Services or its agent; prohibiting the business associate from using or disclosing PHI in any way that would violate the HIPAA Privacy Rule; and prohibiting the business associate from using or disclosing PHI for any purpose other than that described in the contract with the covered entity; and other agreements. But it does not allow the business associate to maintain PHI indefinitely (Rinehart-Thompson 2020b, 250–251).

162. **a** The covered entity may require the individual to make an amendment request in writing and provide a rationale for their amendment request. Such a process must be communicated in advance to the individual (Rinehart-Thompson 2017d, 246–247).

163. d The custodian of health records is the individual who has been designated as having responsibility for the care, custody, control, and proper safekeeping and disclosure of health records for such persons or institutions that prepare and maintain records of healthcare. The custodian of the health record does not have the responsibility or expertise to testify regarding the care of the patient (Brodnik 2017a, 9).

164. b A court order is a document issued by a judge that compels a certain action, such as testimony or the production of documents such as health records. If a document requesting the production of health records is determined to be a court order, it must be complied with regardless of the presence or absence of patient authorization (Rinehart-Thompson 2017a, 58–59).

165. d The process of releasing health record documentation originally created by a different provider is called redisclosure. Federal and state regulations provide specific redisclosure guidelines; however, when in doubt, follow the same principles as the release and disclosure guidelines for other types of health record information (Fahrenholz 2017a, 106).

166. c Healthcare providers with a direct treatment relationship with an individual must provide the notice of privacy practices no later than the date of the first service delivery (for example, first visit to a physician's office, first admission to a hospital, or first encounter at a clinic), including service delivered electronically. Notices must be available at the site where the individual is treated and must be posted in a prominent place where patients can reasonably be expected to read it. If the facility has a website with information on the covered entity's services or benefits, the notice of privacy practices must be prominently posted to it (Rinehart-Thompson 2020b, 260).

167. c A covered entity must act on an individual's request for review of PHI no later than 30 days after the request is made, extending the response period by no more than 30 additional days if it gave the individual a written statement within the 30-day time period explaining the reasons for the delay and the date by which the covered entity will complete its action on the request. The covered entity may extend the time for action on a request for access only once (Rinehart-Thompson 2020b, 255).

168. b The HIPAA Privacy Rule lists two circumstances where protected health information (PHI) can be used or disclosed without the individual's authorization (although the individual must be informed in advance and given an opportunity to agree or object). One of these circumstances is disclosing PHI to a family member or a close friend that is directly relevant to his or her involvement with the patient's care or payment. Likewise, a covered entity may disclose PHI, including the patient's location, general condition, or death, to notify or assist in the notification of a family member, personal representative, or some other person responsible for the patient's care (Rinehart-Thompson 2020b, 265).

169. c Under the Privacy Rule, healthcare providers are not required to obtain patient consent to use or disclose personal identifiable information for treatment, payment, and healthcare operations (Rinehart-Thompson 2020b, 253).

170. b Ownership of the health record has traditionally been granted to the provider who generates the record (Brodnik 2017a, 9).

171. b Confidentiality, as recognized by law and professional codes of ethics, stems from a relationship such as physician and patient, and pertains to the information resulting from that relationship (Brodnik 2017a, 7–8).

172. c A covered entity must act on an individual's request for review of protected health information (PHI) no later than 30 days after the request is made, extending the response period by no more than 30 additional days if it gave the individual a written statement within the 30-day time period explaining the reasons for the delay and the date by which the covered entity will complete its action on the request. The covered entity may extend the time for action on a request for access only once. If PHI is not maintained or located on-site, the covered entity is given within 60 days of receipt to respond to a request (Rinehart-Thompson 2020b, 255).

173. d Covered entities must obtain a written contract with business associates or other entities who handle e-PHI. The written contract must stipulate that the business associate will implement HIPAA administrative, physical, and technical safeguards and procedures and documentation requirements that safeguard the confidentiality, integrity, and availability of the e-PHI that it creates, receives, maintains, or transmits on behalf of the covered entity (Rinehart-Thompson 2020b, 250–251).

174. a Although business associates are not directly regulated by the HIPAA Privacy Rule, they do come under the Privacy Rule's requirements by virtue of their association with one or more covered entities. Some examples of business associates are contract coding professional, billing companies, consultants, accounting firms, and the like (Rinehart-Thompson 2017c, 211).

175. c Hospitals and other healthcare facilities develop health record retention policies to ensure that health records comply with all applicable state and federal regulations, accreditation standards, as well as meet future patient care needs. Most states have established regulations that address how long health records and other healthcare-related documents must be maintained before they can be destroyed (Fahrenholz 2017a, 106–107).

176. c A subpoena *duces tecum* means to bring documents and other records with oneself. Such subpoenas may direct the heath information technology (HIT) professional to bring originals or copies of health records, laboratory reports, x-rays, or other records to a deposition or to court. (Rinehart-Thompson 2020a, 227).

177. a A patient has the opportunity to agree or disagree with being placed in a patient directory. They must be given the opportunity to determine if they want to be placed in the directory or not, but it does not need to be in writing (Rinehart-Thompson 2020b, 264–265).

178. d AHIMA outlines the requirements for the content of the notice of privacy practices. One requirement is that a description (including at least one example) is to be given of the types of uses and disclosures the covered entity is permitted to make for treatment, payment, and healthcare operations (Rinehart-Thompson 2020b, 260–261).

179. a The legal health record is a defined subset of all patient-specific data. The legal health record is the record that will be disclosed upon request by third parties. It includes documentation about health services provided and stored on any media (Fahrenholz 2017c, 50).

180. c Privacy is when a patient has the right to maintain control over certain health information (Rinehart-Thompson 2020b, 248).

181. b Covered entities may disclose PHI to public health entities even if the law does not specifically require the disclosure is for the purpose of preventing or controlling disease; injury; or disability; including, but not limited to, the reporting of disease; injury; vital events such as birth or death; and the conduct of public health surveillance (Brodnik 2017c, 411).

182. **c**   The HIPAA Privacy Rule concept of minimum necessary does not apply to disclosures made for treatment purposes. However, the covered entity must define, within the organization, what information physicians need as part of their treatment role (Thomason 2013, 5).

183. **d**   An individual may revoke an authorization at any time, provided that he or she does so in writing. However, the revocation does not apply when the covered entity has already taken action on the authorization (Rinehart-Thompson 2018, 73).

184. **b**   When entries are made in the health record regarding a patient who is particularly hostile or irritable, general documentation principles apply, such as charting objective facts and avoiding the use of personal opinions, particularly those that are critical of the patient. The degree to which these general principles apply is heightened because a disagreeable patient may cause a provider to use more expressive and inappropriate language. Further, a hostile patient may be more likely to file legal action in the future if the hostility is a personal attribute and not simply a manifestation of his or her medical condition (Rinehart-Thompson 2017b, 179).

185. **a**   The health record may be valuable evidence in a legal proceeding. To be admissible, the court must be confident that the record is complete, accurate, and timely (recorded at the time the event occurred); was documented in the normal course of business; and was made by healthcare providers who have knowledge of the "acts, events, conditions, opinions, or diagnoses appearing in it" (Klaver 2017a, 78–79).

186. **c**   The HIPAA Privacy Rule addresses the issue of personal representatives. Personal representatives are those who are legally authorized to make healthcare decisions on an individual's behalf or to act on behalf of a deceased individual or that individual's estate. Under the Privacy Rule, then, a personal representative must be treated the same as the individual regarding the use and disclosure of the individual's PHI. In this instance, the fact that the sister is listed in the health record as the caregiver does not make her legally authorized as a personal representative under the Privacy Rule. Her request should be refused (Rinehart-Thompson 2017c, 215–216).

187. **c**   The HIPAA Privacy Rule provides only a federal floor, or minimum, on privacy requirements. This means that the federal Privacy Rule does not preempt, or supersede, stricter state statutes (or other federal statutes, for that matter) when they exist (Rinehart-Thompson 2020b, 248–249).

188. **d**   *Security* is the protection of the privacy of individuals and the confidentiality of electronic health records. In other words, security allows only authorized users to access health records. In the broader sense, security also includes the protection of healthcare information from damage, loss, and unauthorized alteration (Brickner 2020b, 286).

189. **a**   Every organization is subject to data security breaches by people from both inside and outside the organization. A data breach is an incident in which an unauthorized individual(s) has potentially viewed, stolen, or used sensitive, protected, or confidential data. Data breaches may involve PHI, personally identifiable information, trade secrets, or intellectual property. In this scenario, the release of employee salary data is information that is usually kept private, it does not meet the definition of HIPAA data breach (Johns 2015, 209)

190. **d**   As part of risk management programs, a "red flag" is used to signal the presence of identity theft (Johns 2015, 221).

191. **d** In order to maintain patient privacy certain audits may need to be completed daily. If a high-profile patient is currently in a facility, for example, access logs may need to be checked daily to determine whether all access to this patient's information by workforce is appropriate (Thomason 2013, 173).

192. **b** The HIPAA Security Rule requires that access to electronic PHI in information systems is monitored. Included in the same standard is the requirement that covered entities examine the activity using access audit logs. Often, they record time stamps that record access and use of the data elements and documents; what was viewed, created, updated, or deleted; the user's identification; the owner of the record; and the physical location on the network where the access occurred. Reviewing the audit trail information would be the first step to identify all employees with the same last name as the patient who have accessed this patient's information (Thomason 2013, 177).

193. **c** Automatic log-off is a security procedure that causes a computer session to end after a predetermined period of inactivity, such as 10 minutes. Multiple software products are available to allow network administrators to set automatic log-off parameters (Reynolds and Brodnik 2017, 277).

194. **d** A legal hold (also known as a preservation order, preservation notice, or litigation hold) suspends the processing or destruction of paper or electronic records. It may be initiated by a court if there is concern that information may be destroyed in cases of current or anticipated litigation, audit, or government investigation. Or it may be initiated by the organization as part of their pre-litigation planning and duty to preserve information in anticipation of litigation (Klaver 2017a, 86–87).

195. **d** A person's right to privacy is the right to be left alone and protected against physical or psychological invasion. It includes freedom from intrusion into one's private affairs to include their healthcare diagnoses (Rinehart-Thompson 2017f, 108–109).

196. **c** Provisions must also be made to protect workstations that are more exposed to the public. For example, locking devices can be used to prevent removal of computer equipment and other devices. Automatic log-outs can be used to prevent access by unauthorized individuals (Brickner 2020b, 300, 311).

197. **d** A strategy included in a good security program is employee security awareness training. Employees are often responsible for threats to data security. Consequently, employee awareness is a particularly important tool in reducing security breaches (Brickner 2020b, 308).

198. **a** A newspaper is not a covered entity under HIPAA. The information also did not come directly from the hospital. The newspaper is not bound by HIPAA and they need not worry that it is committing a HIPAA violation (Rinehart-Thompson 2018, 32–33, 209).

199. **b** A valid authorization has a number of requirements including an expiration date or event. The authorization has to have enough information to identify the patient but it does not specifically have to have the patient account number (Rinehart-Thompson 2020b, 276).

200. **c** The request may be denied in almost all cases, but it cannot be denied for disclosures to a health plan where the individual has paid for a service or item completely out of pocket (Rinehart-Thompson 2020b, 260).

201. a This disclosure of information is a public interest and benefit exception (regarding decedents). As such, written authorization is not required, and it is not a violation of the Privacy Rule. HIPAA consent is optional by nature, so this disclosure is not subject to the HIPAA consent (Rinehart-Thompson 2020b, 266).

202. a Calling a patient by name is subject to the minimum necessary requirement, but it is a permissible incidental disclosure, necessary for the office to conduct its business. It is a disclosure for operational purposes, not payment purposes (Rinehart-Thompson 2020b, 268).

203. d Use is how an organization avails itself of health information internally, as Mary Jane has done in this scenario (Rinehart-Thompson 2020b, 248).

204. d Charles' medical information is protected by the HIPAA Privacy Rule because they have been deceased for more than 50 years (Rinehart-Thompson 2020b, 252).

205. a The requirements for the notice of privacy practices includes a statement that tells the patient to whom they can complain in the event that his or her rights have been violated (Rinehart-Thompson 2020b, 261–262).

206. c In this situation Citizen Bank is not a covered entity and HIPAA does not apply. The bank is also not generating or maintaining identifiable results as this information is being managed directly by the employee health plan (Rinehart-Thompson 2018, 32–33, 210).

207. a The mode is the simplest measure of central tendency. It is used to indicate the most frequent observation in a frequency distribution. The most frequent observation is 30 (Williamson 2020, 407).

208. c The gross death rate is the proportion of all hospital discharges that ended in death. It is the basic indicator of mortality in a healthcare facility. The gross death rate is calculated by dividing the total number of deaths occurring in a given time period by the total number of discharges, including deaths, for the same time period: $25 / 500 = 0.05 \times 100 = 5\%$ (McNeill 2020, 443).

209. d Both x and y axes are in unequal measures, so data are not accurately represented. Line graphs are used to display time trends as opposed to a histogram or bar chart (Williamson 2020, 398).

210. b Line graphs are used to display time trends in data. A line graph is useful for plotting data to make observations. In analyzing the chart, the revenue exceeds the costs (Williamson 2020, 398).

211. d After cases have been identified, extensive information is abstracted from the patients' health records into the registry database or extracted from other databases and automatically entered into the registry database (Sharp 2020, 205).

212. c A dashboard is a visual display of the most important information that a physician would need to see about his patients. These can usually be customized by facility or an individual (White 2020, 264).

213. b Predictive analytics is a branch of data mining concerned with the prediction of future probabilities and trends, also called forecasting (White 2020, 262–263).

214. c   The median is the midpoint of a frequency distribution. It is the point at which 50 percent of observations fall above and 50 percent fall below. Eight is the midpoint of the distribution where 50 percent of the observations fall above and below eight (Williamson 2020, 407).

215. d   A rate is a fraction in which there is a distinct relationship between the numerator and denominator and the denominator often implies a large base population. Coding professional D had the highest absentee rate. In this situation the vacation hours used is added to the sick leave hours used and multiplied by 100 divided by 2,080 hours (for a full time employee). The absentee rate for each employee is calculated as follows: Coding professional A: [(40 + 6) × 100] / 2,080 = 4,600 / 2,080 = 2.21%; Coding professional B: [(22 + 16) × 100] / 2,080 = 3,800 / 2,080 = 1.826 = 1.83%; Coding professional C: [(36 + 8) × 100] / 2,080 = 4,400 / 2,080 = 2.115 = 2.12%; Coding professional D: [(80 + 32) × 100] / 2,080 = 11,200 / 2,080 = 5.38% (White 2020, 24–25).

216. a   Aggregate data include data on groups of people or patients without identifying any particular patient individually. Examples of aggregate data are statistics on the average length of stay (ALOS) for patients discharged within a particular diagnosis-related group (DRG) (Sharp 2020, 199).

217. c   The range is the simplest measure of spread. It is the difference between the smallest and largest values in a frequency distribution (Williamson 2020, 407).

218. a   The mean is the arithmetic average of frequency distribution. Put simply, it is the sum of all the values in a frequency distribution divided by the frequency: (10 + 15 + 20 + 25 + 25) / 5 = 19 (Williamson 2020, 406).

219. a   A table should contain all the information the user needs to understand the data in it. All tables should include the following elements: the table legend or title; column titles; the body of the table, which includes actual data; lines that divide certain parts of the table; and a footnote or reference citation if the table text was take from an article or other source. This table is missing the title (Williamson 2020, 393–394).

220. c   Length of stay (LOS) is calculated for each patient after he or she is discharged from the hospital. It is the number of calendar days from the day of patient admission to the day of discharge (31 − 21) + 1 = 11 days (McNeill 2020, 440).

221. d   Internal users of secondary data are individuals located within the healthcare facility. Internal users include medical staff and administrative and management staff. Secondary data enable these users to identify patterns and trends that are helpful in patient care, long-term planning, budgeting, and benchmarking with other facilities (Sharp 2020, 199).

222. c   The gross autopsy rate is the proportion or percentage of deaths that are followed by the performance of autopsy. In this case, (5 / 25) × 100 = 20% (McNeill 2020, 446).

223. d   A pie chart is an easily understood chart in which the sizes of the slices of the pie show the proportional contribution of each part. Pie charts can be used to show the component parts of a single group or variable (Williamson 2020, 397–398).

224. d   The result of the official count taken at midnight is the daily inpatient census. This is the number of inpatients present at the official census-taking time each day. Also included in the daily inpatient census are any patients who were admitted and discharged the same day (McNeill 2020, 436).

225. **a** The average length of stay (ALOS) is calculated from the total length of stay (LOS). The total LOS divided by the number of patients discharged is the ALOS (McNeill 2020, 441).

226. **c** The gross death rate is the proportion of all hospital discharges that ended in death. It is the basic indicator of mortality in a healthcare facility. The gross death rate is calculated by dividing the total number of deaths occurring in a given time period by the total number of discharges, including deaths, for the same time period (McNeill 2020, 443).

227. **a** A unit of measure that reflects the services received by one inpatient during a 24-hour period is an inpatient service day (IPSD). The number of inpatient service days for a 24-hour period is equal to the daily inpatient census, that is, one service day for each patient treated (McNeill 2020, 436).

228. **b** The census reports patient activity for a 24-hour reporting period. Included in the census report are the number of inpatients admitted and discharged for the previous 24-hour period and the number of intrahospital transfers (McNeill 2020, 436).

229. **c** An incidence rate is used to compare the frequency of disease in different populations. Populations are compared using rates instead of raw numbers because rates adjust for differences in population size. The incidence rate is the probability or risk of illness in a population over a period of time (McNeill 2020, 464).

230. **b** External data sources refers to data collected outside an organization. For example, a census, reports from the Centers for Medicare and Medicaid Services (CMS) or the Centers for Disease Control (CDC), economic databases, journals, even social media have links to outside data (White 2020, 262).

231. **a** The Medicare Provider Analysis and Review (MEDPAR) file is made up of acute-care hospital and skilled nursing facility (SNF) claims data for all Medicare claims. The MEDPAR file is frequently used for research on topics such as charges for particular types of care and MS-DRGs. The limitation of the MEDPAR data for research purposes is that the file contains only Medicare patients (Sharp 2020, 211).

232. **b** A rate is a fraction in which there is a distinct relationship between the numerator and denominator and the denominator often implies a large base population. Add each employee's sick leave hours together to get a total of 102. Multiplying 2,080 (full time equivalent) by 5 (number of employees) equals 10,400. Take the total sick leave hours (102) and multiply by 100, then divide it by the total hours for the five full time employees (10,400). Calculations: $(6 + 16 + 8 + 32 + 40) = 102$ hours total sick leave time; $(2,080 \times 5) = 10,400$ total hours for the five coding professionals; $(102 \times 100) / 10,400 = 10,200 / 10,400 = 0.98\%$ total sick leave rate (White 2020, 24–25).

233. **a** The geometric mean length of stay (GMLOS) is the nth root of a series of n length of stays. For example, if there are five length of stay (LOS) data points, multiply the LOS data points together, and then take the 5th root of the product. The GMLOS is less influenced by large outliers than the AMLOS and, therefore, is a good measure of the center of the distribution (Casto and White 2021, 74).

234. **c** Geographic practice cost index (GPCI) is the number used to multiply each RVU so that it better reflects a geographical area's relative costs. The practice expense GPCI is higher in Seattle at 1.098 (Casto and White 2021, 123).

235. **b** Length of stay (LOS) is calculated for each patient after he or she is discharged from the hospital. It is the number of calendar days from the day of patient admission to the day of discharge. When the patient is admitted and discharged in the same month, the LOS is determined by subtracting the date of admission from the date of discharge (McNeill 2020, 440).

236. **d** The unique identifier in the patient table is the patient number. It is unique to each patient. Patient last name, first name, and date of birth can be shared with other patients, but the identifier will not be shared (Sayles and Kavanaugh-Burke 2021, 50).

237. **a** As opposed to periodic and exception reports, demand reports, also known as ad hoc reports, are produced as needed, whenever a manager demands or asks for it. Usually, demand reports are produced through report generators or database query languages and are customized by the manager (Johns 2015, 236).

238. **c** When doing external benchmarking, the other organizations need not be in the same region of the country, but they should be comparable in terms of patient mix and size. The data from the two hospitals are not comparable because Hospital A discharges more patients than Hospital B. In addition, data on the comparability of severity of illness between the two hospitals is lacking and an informed decision cannot be made (Shaw and Carter 2019, 42).

239. **b** A pie chart is used to show the relationship of each part to the whole, in other words, how each part contributes to the total product or process. The 360 degrees of the circle, or pie, represent the total, or 100 percent. The pie is divided into "slices" proportionate to each component's percentage of the whole. Review of the pie chart shows that the emergency department has had significant patient growth over the two-year period. By using this patient profile data for performance improvement, the hospital should examine capacity changes for this department (Shaw and Carter 2019, 86–87).

240. **c** The medical staff department is particularly interested in the ICD-10-CM codes associated with each physician. Because diagnostic codes can identify untoward events that occur during hospitalization, the quality of a physician's services can be identified through reports called physician reappointment summaries. These summaries outline the number of cases by diagnosis and procedure type, LOS, and infection and mortality statistics. At reappointment to a facility's medical staff, code-based reports are required. The medical staff department accumulates these reports and works with the elected or appointed medical staff leadership to ensure that a thorough analysis of each physician's activities takes place before he or she is reappointed to the staff (Schraffenberger and Kuehn 2011, 443).

241. **c** Family practice has the largest variance with the potential for the most savings (Prater 2020, 630).

242. **b** Reading this graph, the full-time coding professional productivity is higher than part-time coding professional productivity. The cause for this difference must be identified before any solution can be developed to increase the productivity of the part-time coding professionals (Prater 2020, 629–630).

243. **a** The data on the graph shows the current system is generating more projected cost savings on a monthly basis than the e-WebCoding system. Learning to use data analysis tools and data aggregation techniques is important for improvement decisions. Making decisions based on actual experience and aggregate data is much better than making decisions based on intuition or gut feelings (Shaw and Carter 2019, 89–90).

244. d   Medicaid charges are larger than the charges to commercial insurance and TRICARE; however, the facility receives a smaller payment from Medicaid. There is an adjustment of 36 percent, meaning that the facility had to adjust their charges 36 percent from the actual amount billed and the amount they receive in payment (Williamson 2020, 394).

245. b   The Medicare Provider Analysis and Review (MEDPAR) file is made up of acute-care hospital and SNF claims data for all Medicare claims. The MEDPAR file is frequently used for research on topics such as charges for particular types of care and DRGs. The limitation of the MEDPAR data for research purposes is that the file contains only Medicare patients (Sharp 2020, 211).

246. b   A gross autopsy rate is the proportion or percentage of deaths that are followed by the performance of autopsy (McNeill 2020, 446).

247. c   Pie charts are best to use when you want to show each category's percentage of the total. They do not show changes over time. A circle is divided into sections such as wedges or slices. These represent percentages of the total (100 percent) (White 2020, 212–213).

248. a   To determine the case-mix index, take the sum of all relative weights and divide by the total number of discharges. The formula for computing case-mix is: The sum of the weights of MS-DRGs for patients discharged during a given period divided by the total number of patients discharged (McNeill 2020, 451).

249. c   C-section rate: $(101 \times 100) / 504 = 10,100 / 504 = 20.039 = 20.04\%$ (White 2020, 134–135).

250. a   Descriptive analytics describe raw data. This type of analytics is useful because it helps us see what was done in the past. We can learn from our past behaviors and begin to look at how we can effect some change in the future. Most of the statistics used in healthcare fall into this category. This type of analytics is used to understand at an aggregate level what is happening with patients in healthcare facilities (White 2020, 261–262).

251. d   Unlike retrospective analytical tools, such as predictive modeling, real-time analytics refers to data that can be accessed as they come into a computer system. Real-time analytics, also referred to as streaming analytics, implies instantaneous results; however, the data may not be immediately available, but rather available within a few minutes. The most valuable data in this category are those that are collected and analyzed during the customer interaction, not the review afterward (White 2020, 264).

252. a   A proportion is a type of ratio in which x is a portion of the whole $(x + y)$. In a proportion, the numerator is always included in the denominator. $182 / 270 = 0.67$ (White 2020, 23).

253. c   All states have a health department with a division that is required to track and record communicable diseases. When a patient is diagnosed with one of the diseases from the health department's communicable disease list, the healthcare organization must notify the public health department. Measles usually requires reporting within 24 hours of a suspected diagnosis to the public health department. The other three need to be reported, but only within three working days of identification (Shaw and Carter 2019, 177–178).

254. b   Inferential statistics help make inferences or guesses about a larger group of data by drawing conclusions from a small group of data (White 2020, 3).

255. b   Predictive modeling is a process used in predictive analysis to identify patterns that can be used to determine the odds of a particular outcome based on the observed data. That is, statistics from the past are reviewed to determine what is likely to happen in the future. Predictive modeling is used by many companies that want to predict future trends (White 2020, 263–264).

256. c   Secondary data sources are data derived from primary sources and may be collected by someone other than the primary user. Secondary data sources are facility specific. The physician index is an example of a secondary data source (White 2020, 4–5).

257. c   The result of the official count taken at midnight is the daily inpatient census (McNeill 2020, 436).

258. c   Relations are established in a relational database by the primary key of one table becoming a foreign key in another table. In this case, the patient number is the primary key in the patient table and used as the foreign key in the visit table (Johns 2015, 127–128).

259. a   Case finding is a method used to identify the patients who have been seen or treated in the facility for the particular disease or condition of interest to the registry. After cases have been identified, extensive information is abstracted from the patients' paper-based health records into the registry database or extracted from other databases and automatically entered into the registry database (Sharp 2020, 201).

260. c   Comparative data uses aggregate data to describe the experiences of unique types of patients with one or more aspects of their care (Shaw and Carter 2019, 348).

261. a   Healthcare facilities are interested in births and deaths, fetal deaths, and induced terminations of pregnancy; facilities generally are responsible for completing certificates for births, fetal deaths, abortions, and occasionally deaths. All states have laws that require this data. The certificates are reported to the individual state registrars and maintained permanently. State vital statistics registrars compile the data and report them to the NCHS (White 2020, 3–4).

262. b   The case fatality rate is the total number of deaths due to a specific illness during a given time period divided by the total number of cases during the same period. (3 × 100) / 58 = 300 / 58 = 5.17% (White 2020, 88–89).

263. c   After trauma cases have been identified, information is abstracted from the health records of the injured patients and entered into the trauma registry database (Sharp 2020, 204–205).

264. c   The lead coding professional's annual salary is $20.35 × 2,080 (hours per year) = $42,328. The lead coding professional's productivity is 7.5 hours per day × 4 records per hour = 30 records per day. 30 records per day × 5 days per week × 52 weeks per year = 7,800 records per year. Yearly salary of $42,328 / 7,800 records per year = $5.43 per record (White 2020, 148).

265. d   A table is an orderly arrangement of values that groups data into rows and columns. Almost any type of quantitative information can be grouped into tables. Columns allow you to read data up and down, and rows allow you to read data across. The columns and rows should be labeled. In this table, the physician with the lowest rate of deficiency is number 637 (White 2020, 198–199).

266. c   A proportion is a particular type of ratio in which x is a portion of the whole ($x + y$) (McNeill 2020, 433).

267. **d** Healthcare data are divided into two broad categories of quantitative and qualitative data. Quantitative data are numeric while qualitative data describe observations. Quantitative data can be numerically counted. They deal with measurements (White 2020, 262).

268. **c** A table is an orderly arrangement of values that groups data into rows and columns. Almost any type of quantitative information can be grouped into tables. Columns allow you to read data up and down, and rows allow you to read data across. The columns and rows should be labeled. In this table, personal mobile device has the highest percent of physicians using the system (White 2020, 198–199).

269. **d** The HIPAA Security Rule requires that access to electronic PHI in information systems is monitored. Included in the same standard is the requirement that covered entities examine the activity using access audit logs. Often they record time stamps that record access and use of the data elements and documents; what was viewed, created, updated, or deleted; the user's identification; the owner of the record; and the physical location on the network where the access occurred. Reviewing the audit trail information would be the first step in identifying all employees who have accessed this patient's information (Thomason 2013, 177).

270. **a** A rate is a fraction in which there is a distinct relationship between the numerator and denominator and the denominator often implies a large base population. (67 / 150) × 100 = 44.66 = 44.7% (White 2020, 24–25).

271. **d** Scatter diagrams are used to plot the points for two continuous variables that may be related to each other in some way. For example, one might want to look at whether age and blood pressure are related. One variable, age, would be plotted on the vertical axis of the graph, and the other variable, blood pressure, would be plotted on the horizontal axis (Williamson 2020, 399).

272. **c** A table is an orderly arrangement of values that groups data into rows and columns. Almost any type of quantitative information can be grouped into tables. Columns allow you to read data up and down, and rows allow you to read data across. The columns and rows should be labeled. In this table, the payment source with the highest denial rate is Worker's Compensation (White 2020, 198–199).

273. **d** Vaginal delivery rate: (403 × 100) / 504 = 40,300 / 504 = 79.96% (White 2020, 134–135).

274. **d** It is a requirement of the HIPAA Security Rule to implement ways that document access to information systems that contain electronic PHI. One of the ways to do this is to review the individuals that have viewed, created, updated, or deleted information within a health record. In this instance the privacy officer should review this information to determine if the patient complaint is valid (Thomason 2013, 177).

275. **b** A table is an orderly arrangement of values that groups data into rows and columns. Almost any type of quantitative information can be grouped into tables. Columns allow you to read data up and down, and rows allow you to read data across. The columns and rows should be labeled. In order to determine the amount of time it will take to reconcile all of the denials the number of denials is multiplied by the amount of time it takes to complete each denial (1.5 hours). 1.5 hours × 176 denials = 264 hours (White 2020, 198–199).

276. **a** A bed count, also called an inpatient bed count, is the number of available hospital inpatient beds, both occupied and vacant, on any given day. Temporary beds are not included in the bed count for percentage of occupancy (White 2020, 52).

277. **b** Healthcare facilities have a census, which is the count of patients present at a specific time and in a particular place (White 2020, 4).

278. **a** The ratio of a part to the whole is often expressed as a percentage. Percentages are a useful way to make fair comparisons. The percentage of physicians not using the system is 2.2%. (11 physicians not using the system × 100) / 500 = 1,100 / 500 = 2.2% (White 2020, 16–17).

279. **b** When analyzing this table one is able to determine that 1.22 is the lowest relative value unit (RVU) (Williamson 2020, 394).

280. **d** The new graduate coding professional's salary is $15.50 × 2,080 (hours per year) = $32,240. Productivity is 7.5 hours per day × 3 records per hour = 22.5 records per day. 22.5 records × 5 days per week × 52 weeks per year = 5,850 records per year. $32,240 / 5,850 = $5.51 per record (White 2020, 148).

281. **c** Prescriptive analytics is a field of analytics that allows users to prescribe a number of different possible actions. This type of analytics predicts what will happen, but also provides recommendations that will take advantage of the predictions (White 2020, 264).

282. **d** A review of the distribution between MS-DRG triples, pairs, and singles against patient record documentation would provide information to support coding and billing of appropriate CCs and MCCs. The appropriateness of assigning CCs and MCCs will impact the organization's case-mix index and must be monitored. The CMI is a measure of the average revenue received per case. Many hospitals closely monitor the movement of their CMI for inpatient populations for which payment is based on DRGs (Gordon, M. L. 2020, 493).

283. **d** When an incomplete record is not rectified within a specific number of days as indicated in the medical staff rules and regulations, the record is considered to be a delinquent record. Generally, an incomplete record is considered delinquent after it has been available to the physician for completion for 15 to 30 days. This question does not provide enough information on the standard as the medical staff rules and regulations on delinquent records are not defined (Sayles 2020b, 77).

284. **a** Normalization is breaking the data elements into the level of detail desired by the healthcare facility (Sayles and Kavanaugh-Burke 2021, 49).

285. **d** Descriptive analytics use a group of statistical techniques to describe data such as means, frequency distributions, and is used to describe the characteristics of a specific group or population (Sayles and Kavanaugh-Burke 2021, 36).

286. **a** Inter-reliability measures the reproducibility of the measurement of a data point between two raters (White 2021, 21–22).

287. **a** The postoperative mortality rate refers to the number of deaths occurring after an operation has been performed. 1/32 = 0.03125 or 3.13% (White 2020, 91–92).

288. **c** The telephone appointments would cost $875.00; $3.50 × 250 = $875.00 (White 2020, 152).

289. **b** The email appointments would cost $375.00; $1.50 × 250 = $375.00 (White 2020, 152).

290. c   To calculate the cost savings $875.00 − $375.00 = $500.00 (White 2020, 152).

291. d   Prescriptive analytics uses information generated from descriptive and predictive analytics and modeling to determine a strategy for the best outcome or to suggest a course of action to solve a problem. Once the COVID-19 pandemic slows or ends, prescriptive analytics will be used to improve the preparation and mitigation efforts that government and healthcare organizations must do to lessen the impact of the next pandemic (Sayles and Kavanaugh-Burke 2021, 36).

292. a   In the "rate of unapproved abbreviations" column, physician #802 has the highest rate of unapproved abbreviations (25.6 percent), which is higher than any other physician (Williamson 2020, 394).

293. d   In the "# of unapproved abbreviations" column physician #102 has the highest number of unapproved abbreviations (34), which is higher than any other physician (Williamson 2020, 394).

294. c   The total rate of unapproved abbreviations is calculated by taking the # of unapproved abbreviation divided by the # of discharges × 100. (140/1187) × 100 = 11.8% (Williamson 2020, 394).

295. d   This is calculated: 9,000 / (100 × 5) = 9,000 / 500 = 18 FTEs. The number of FTEs will be the total number of patients divided by the total number of records required per week (assuming a five-day workweek) (White 2020, 157–158).

296. b   One standard deviation from the mean = 68.26 percent of the area, two standard deviations = 95.45 percent of the area, and three standard deviations = 99.74 percent of the area under the curve (Williamson 2020, 408–409).

297. b   Diagnostic analytics helps a healthcare organization determine why something happened. Diagnostic analytics tools such as dashboards and data mining are performed (Sayles and Kavanaugh-Burke 2021, 36).

298. a   A Pareto chart can help analyze data about the frequency or causes of problems in a process. In this scenario, the healthcare organization can use the Pareto to graphically display why patients are being admitted to the hospital. This data can then be used to reduce the number of admissions (Williamson 2020, 397).

299. d   Utilization review assesses the appropriateness of the setting for the healthcare service in the continuum of care and the level of service. Patients' severity of illness and other medical conditions and illnesses are also factored in (Casto and White 2021, 28–29).

300. a   Present on admission (POA) is defined as a condition present at the time the order for inpatient admission occurs—conditions that develop during an outpatient encounter, including the emergency department, observation, or outpatient surgery, are considered as present on admission. A POA indicator is assigned to principal and secondary diagnoses and the external cause of injury codes based on physician documentation. The POA indicator is used to determine if a healthcare-acquired condition has occurred. If the healthcare-acquired condition has occurred this will negatively impact the hospital reimbursement for this claim (Gordon, M. L. 2020, 489).

301. c A comorbid condition is a condition that existed at admission and will likely cause an increase in the patient's length stay. Diabetes existed at the time of admission and is a comorbid condition (Schraffenberger and Palkie 2022, 92–93).

302. a Unbundling is the practice of using multiple codes that describe individual components of a procedure rather than an appropriate single code that describes all steps of the procedure performed. Unbundling can result in the healthcare organization receiving an overpayment and is considered abuse as it violates coding guidelines. The coding professional should be counseled to stop this practice immediately (Foltz and Lankisch 2020, 500).

303. d National Correct Coding Initiative (NCCI) is a predefined set of edits created by Medicare to prevent improper payment when incorrect code combinations are reported. The NCCI contains two types of edits, one of which are mutually exclusive edits that consist of code pairs that should not be reported together for a number of reasons (Casto and White 2021, 216–217).

304. b Medicare inpatients are reimbursed through MS-DRGs calculated for each hospital encounter. These are assigned with the help of a grouper (Sayles 2020b, 87; Gordon, M. L. 2020, 493).

305. c When calculating case mix using MS-DRGs, the case-mix index (CMI) is the average relative weight of all cases treated at a given facility or by a given physician, which reflects the resource intensity or clinical severity of a specific group in relation to the other groups in the classification system. The calculation for this data set is 33.3016 / 30 = 1.110 (Gordon, M. L. 2020, 493–494).

306. c A query may not be appropriate because the clinical information or clinical picture does not appear to support the documentation of a condition or procedure. In situations where the provider's documented diagnosis does not appear to be supported by clinical findings, a healthcare entity's policies can provide guidance on a process for addressing the issue without querying the attending physician (Brinda 2020, 186–187).

307. c Signs and symptoms integral to the disease process should not be coded. In this case the fever, chest pain, and cough are integral to the pneumonia. The specific type of pneumonia would be coded based on the documentation of staph (Schraffenberger and Palkie 2022, 35).

308. d During surgery, physicians may take some normal-looking skin around the growth. Removal of the normal-looking skin is known as taking margins. This is done to be sure no cancer cells are left behind. The total size of the excised area, including margins, is needed for accurate coding. Usually, this information is provided in the operative report (Smith 2021, 77–78).

309. a Inpatient hospitals were required to submit POA information on diagnoses for inpatient Medicare discharges (Gordon, M. L. 2020, 489).

310. d Signs and symptoms integral to the disease process should not be coded. In this case the nausea, vomiting, and abdominal pain are integral to the acute cholecystitis (Schraffenberger and Palkie 2022, 35).

311. b The principal diagnosis is designated and defined as the condition established after study chiefly responsible for occasioning the admission of the patient to the hospital for care. The abdominal pain would not be coded as it is a symptom of the gastroenteritis (Schraffenberger and Palkie 2022, 95).

312. **c** As a result of the disparity in documentation practices by providers, querying has become a common communication and educational method to advocate proper documentation practices. Queries can be made in situations when there is clinical evidence for a higher degree of specificity or severity (Brinda 2020, 186–187).

313. **d** Upcoding is the practice of using a code that results in a higher payment to the provider that actually reflects the service of item provided (Foltz and Lankisch 2020, 500).

314. **c** The principal diagnosis is designated and defined as the condition established after study chiefly responsible for occasioning the admission of the patient to the hospital for care (Schraffenberger and Palkie 2022, 95).

315. **a** A complex repair of a wound goes beyond layer closure and involves at least one of the following: exposure of bone, cartilage, tendon, or named neurovascular structure; debridement or wound edges; extensive undermining; involvement of free margins of helical rim, vermilion border, or nostril rim; or placement of retention sutures (Huey 2021, 82).

316. **c** A patient may have a history of a primary site of malignancy but later develops a secondary neoplasm or a metastatic site at another location. When this occurs, the treatment is likely to be directed to the secondary site. The secondary site code is assigned first with a category Z85 code used as an additional diagnosis code (Schraffenberger and Palkie 2022, 151–152).

317. **a** In the unusual instance when two or more diagnoses equally meet the criteria for principal diagnosis, as determined by the circumstances of admission, diagnostic workup, or the therapy provided, and the Alphabetic Index, Tabular List, or another coding guideline does not provide sequencing in such cases, any one of the diagnoses may be sequenced first (Schraffenberger and Palkie 2022, 96).

318. **b** The Excludes1 note is found in the Tabular List. The Excludes1 note indicates that the conditions listed after it cannot ever be used at the same time as the code above the Excludes1 note. The benign neoplasm on the vermillion border of the lip (D10.0) is not coded in category D23 (Schraffenberger and Palkie 2022, 27–28).

319. **c** The patient has the signs and symptoms and responded to treatment that would be given because of asthma with status asthmaticus. The physician can be queried based on the clinical indicators of a diagnosis when no documentation of the condition is present (Schraffenberger and Palkie 2022, 360; Brinda 2020, 186–187).

320. **d** Certain ICD-10-CM categories have applicable seventh characters. The applicable seventh character is required for all codes within the category, or as the notes in the Tabular List instruct. The seventh character must always be the seventh character in the data field. If a code that requires a seventh character does not contain six characters, a placeholder X must be used to fill in the empty characters (Schraffenberger and Palkie 2022, 20–21).

321. **b** Signs, symptoms, abnormal test results, or other reasons for the outpatient visit are used when a physician qualifies a diagnostic statement as "possible," "probable," "suspected," "questionable," "rule out," or "working diagnosis," or other similar terms indicating uncertainty (Schraffenberger and Palkie 2022, 105).

322. **a** This patient's sepsis has resolved before being admitted to the hospital and would be considered a previous condition. She is treated with an aspiration dilation and curettage with products of conception found. The patient's principal diagnosis would be the miscarriage (Schraffenberger and Palkie 2022, 95, 509–510).

323. **a** The appropriateness of assigning CCs and MCCs will impact the organization's case-mix index and must be monitored. The CMI is a measure of the average revenue received per case. Many hospitals closely monitor the movement of their CMI for inpatient populations for which payment is based on DRGs (Gordon, M. L. 2020, 493).

324. **b** Sepsis is a serious medical condition caused by the body's immune response to an infection. Coding guideline I.C.1.e tells us that code A41.01 is for sepsis with methicillin-susceptible *Staphylococcus aureus*. Because abdominal pain is a symptom of diverticulitis, only the diverticulitis of the colon is coded (Schraffenberger and Palkie 2022, 35, 119–120).

325. **d** Status indicator code T for APC 0044 designates that the APC payment is subject to payment reduction when multiple procedures are performed during the same visit. In this case, there were no additional procedures, so the status indicator does not affect payment (Casto and White 2021, 109–110).

326. **a** Diabetes would be referenced in the Index, subterm Type I, with gangrene, which directs the coding professional to E10.52 (Schraffenberger and Palkie 2022, 43–44).

327. **d** Assign codes to their highest level of specificity. Diagnosis is of eyelid, D23.111 is the correct code (Schraffenberger and Palkie 2022, 43–44).

328. **d** Modifiers are appended to the code to provide more information or alert the payer that a payment change is required. Modifier 55 is used to identify that the physician provided only postoperative care services for a particular procedure (Huey 2021, 54, 57).

329. **d** Begin with the main term Revision; pacemaker site; chest (Huey 2021, 24).

330. **a** To determine the appropriate MS-DRG, a claim for a healthcare encounter is first classified into 1 of 25 major diagnostic categories, or MDCs. The principal diagnosis determines the MDC assignment (Casto and White 2021, 76).

331. **b** Begin with the main term Biopsy, artery, temporal (Huey 2021, 24).

332. **b** The root operation Drainage is defined as taking, or letting out fluids and/or gases from a body part. The value of 9 is used for Drainage. Examples are incision and drainage and arthrotomy for fluid drainage (Kuehn and Jorwic 2021, 85).

333. **b** Z21, Asymptomatic HIV infection status is to be used when the patient without any documentation of symptoms is listed as being "HIV positive," "known HIV," "HIV test positive," or similar terminology. Do not use this code if the term "AIDS" is used or if the patient is treated for any HIV-related illness or is described as having any condition(s) resulting from HIV positive status; use B20 in these cases (ICD-10-CM Coding Guideline I.C.1.a.2.d.; Schraffenberger and Palkie 2022, 114).

334. **d** Utilization review is the process to determine if medical care meets objective screening criteria (Miller 2020, 55).

335. **d** CMS established the hospital-acquired conditions provision in the acute-care inpatient setting as part of its value-based purchasing program (Casto and White 2021, 71–72, 85–86).

336. a   Coinsurance refers to the amount the insured pays as a requirement of the insurance policy. The coinsurance amount is $85 \times 0.20 = $17. A $15 copay is lower than the 20 percent ($17) coinsurance (Gordon, M. L. 2020, 478).

337. d   Principal diagnosis is defined as the condition which, after study, is determined to have occasioned the admission of the patient to the hospital for care (Schraffenberger and Palkie 2022, 92).

338. b   Each base Medicare severity diagnosis-related group (MS-DRG) can be subdivided in one of three possible alternatives: Major Complication/Comorbidity (MCC); Complication/Comorbidity (CC); and Non-CC (Gordon, M. L. 2020, 493).

339. a   Present on admission (POA) is defined as a condition present at the time the order for inpatient admission occurs—conditions that develop during an outpatient encounter, including the emergency department, observation, or outpatient surgery, are considered as present on admission. A POA indicator is assigned to principal and secondary diagnoses and the external cause of injury codes (Gordon, M. L. 2020, 489).

340. a   The root operation Performance is used to code the mechanical ventilation for greater than 96 hours. Section—Extracorporeal Assistance and Performance—character 5; Physiological Systems—character A; Root Operation is Performance—character 1; Body System is Respiratory—character 9; Duration is greater than 96 hours—character 5; Function Value Ventilation—character 5; and No Qualifier—character Z (Kuehn and Jorwic 2021, 443–444).

341. d   The error rates are not comparable because there is no data about the number of records coded during the period by each coding professional (Schraffenberger and Kuehn 2011, 319–320).

342. b   CMS implemented the National Correct Coding Initiative (NCCI) in 1996 to develop correct coding methodologies to improve the appropriate payment of Medicare Part B claims (Casto and White 2021, 216–217).

343. c   The HIM department can plan focused reviews based on specific problem areas after the initial baseline review has been completed. This would be called a focused review (Foltz and Lankisch 2020, 513–514).

344. b   Unbundling refers to a billing practice in which providers use multiple procedure codes for a group of procedures instead of the appropriate combination code (Foltz and Lankisch 2020, 500).

345. a   For established patients, the requirements differ depending on the level of service. Code 99211 does not require a history, examination, medical decision-making, or presence of a physician (Huey 2021, 343).

346. c   An explanation of benefits is a report sent from a healthcare insurer to the policyholder and to the provider that describes the healthcare service, its cost, applicable cost sharing, and the amount the healthcare insurer will cover. The reminder is the policyholder's responsibility (Casto and White 2021, 172).

347. a   Outpatient coding guidelines do not allow coding of possible conditions as a diagnosis for the patient. Do not code diagnoses documented as "probable," "suspected," "questionable," "rule out," or "working diagnosis," or other similar terms indicating uncertainty. Rather, code the condition(s) to the highest degree of certainty for that encounter or visit, such as symptoms, signs, abnormal test results, or other reason for the visit (Huey 2021, 29).

348. c   A bronchoscopy with brushings and washings is considered a diagnostic bronchoscopy and not a biopsy. Code 31623 specifies brushings, and 31622 is selected for washings (Huey 2021, 113–114).

349. b   The NCCI edits (which most providers have built into their claims software) explain what procedures and services cannot be billed together on the same day of service for a patient. The mutually exclusive edit applies to improbable or impossible combinations of codes (Casto and White 2021, 216–217).

350. b   A hospital-acquired condition (HAC) is a select group of reasonably preventable conditions for which hospitals should not receive additional payment when one of the conditions was not present on admission (POA) (Gordon, M. L. 2020, 489).

351. c   Treatment and anatomic location are not factors in the sequencing of burn conditions. Code all burns with the highest degree of burn sequenced first (Schraffenberger and Palkie 2022, 586).

352. d   Training provides new or current employees with knowledge, skills, and abilities related to specific competencies needed to perform their current job. Coding education must be provided in this situation in order to improve the accuracy of principal diagnosis assignment. Accurate assignment of principal diagnosis is a critical part of the inpatient coding process as this assignment has direct impact on the MS-DRG assignment (Casto and White 2021, 78, 189–191; Prater 2020, 643–644).

353. a   AIDS stands for acquired immunodeficiency syndrome, frequently called human immunodeficiency infection (HIV). According to coding guideline I.C.1.a.(2)(a), when a patient is treated for a complication associated with HIV infection, the B20 code is assigned as the principal diagnosis, followed by the code for the complication. Patients who are admitted for an HIV-related illness should be assigned a minimum of two codes in the following order: B20 to identify the HIV disease and additional codes to identify other diagnoses (Schraffenberger and Palkie 2022, 113–114).

354. b   If the treatment is directed at the malignancy, designate the malignancy as the first-listed diagnosis. The only exception to this guideline is if a patient admission or encounter is for the purpose of radiotherapy, immunotherapy, or chemotherapy. When the purpose of the encounter or hospital admission is for radiotherapy, or for antineoplastic chemotherapy, use the Z code as the first-listed diagnosis (Schraffenberger and Palkie 2022, 147).

355. a   Discharged, not final billed (DNFB) refers to accounts where the patient has been discharged but the charges have not been processed or billed (Casto and White 2021, 188).

356. a   The NCCI edits (which most providers have built into their claims software) explain what procedures and services cannot be billed together on the same day of service for a patient. The medically unlikely edit applies to improbable or impossible combinations of codes (Casto and White 2021, 216–217).

357. d   When the claim is submitted, the reviewer should compare all the diagnoses and procedures included on the bill with the coded information in the health record system. This process will help identify whether the communication software between the health record system and the billing system is functioning correctly. The HIM department should share the results of this comparison with patient financial services and the information technology department (Schraffenberger and Kuehn 2011, 320).

358. **d** A CDI program provides a mechanism for the coding staff to communicate with the physician regarding nonspecific diagnostic statements or when additional diagnoses are suspected but not clearly stated in the record, which helps to avoid assumption coding (Schraffenberger and Kuehn 2011, 356).

359. **d** It is not appropriate for the coding professional to assume that the removal was done by either snare or hot biopsy forceps. The coding professional must query the physician to assign the appropriate code (Brinda 2020, 186).

360. **c** This is an example of a normal delivery, full-term, single, healthy liveborn infant with an episiotomy. No other procedures or manipulation needed to aid in delivery. The Z3A code is used to indicate the 40 weeks of gestation of the pregnancy. The correct ICD-10-PCS procedure code is 0W8NXZZ, division of the female perineum (Schraffenberger and Palkie 2022, 496; Kuehn and Jorwic 2021, 146).

361. **a** CMS established the hospital-acquired conditions provision in the acute-care inpatient setting as part of its value-based purchasing program (Casto and White 2021, 71–72, 85–86).

362. **b** External cause of injury codes provide a means to classify environmental events, circumstances, and conditions as the cause of injury, poisoning, and other adverse effects. These codes are used in addition to codes from other chapters of ICD-10-CM; in this case the external cause code for fall from a curb is used to describe how the patient was injured (Schraffenberger and Palkie 2022, 639).

363. **a** Per CPT Coding Guidelines, when a planned procedure is terminated prior to completed for cause, the intended procedure is coded with a modifier. Because general anesthesia was used, modifier 74 is appropriate in this case (Smith 2021, 55).

364. **c** A healthcare entity's query policy should address the question of whom to query. The query is directed to the provider who originated the progress note or other report in question. This could include the attending physician, consulting physician, or the surgeon. In most cases, a query for abnormal test results would be directed to the attending physician (Brinda 2020, 186–187).

365. **d** Healthcare Common Procedure Coding System (HCPCS) Level II codes were developed by CMS for use in reporting health services not covered in CPT. Level II codes are provided for injectable drugs, ambulance services, prosthetic devices, and selected providers services. Crutches are classified as durable medical equipment and would be coded with a HCPCS Level II code (Smith 2021, 6).

366. **b** It is recommended that the healthcare entity's policy address the query format. A query generally includes the following information: patient name, admission date or date of service, health record number, account number, date query initiated, name and contact information of the individual initiating the query, and statement of the issue in the form of a question along with clinical indicators specified from the chart (for example, history and physical states urosepsis, lab reports WBC of 14,400, emergency department report fever of 102°F) (Brinda 2020, 186).

367. **c** The heart catheterization is a percutaneous approach to the circulatory system of the body, not a definitive procedure. Code the actual root operations or root types that were performed through the catheter. In this case, the diagnostic test of heart catheterization was the percutaneous approach to the circulatory system of the body to take sampling and pressure measurements. The root operation would be measurement (Kuehn and Jorwic 2021, 226).

368. **b**   Codes 88302–88309 are assigned based on the specific specimen examined. The type of specimen included in each code is listed alphabetically under the code. A kidney biopsy specimen examination, both gross and microscopic, is coded to 88305 (Huey 2021, 251).

369. **a**   Medical visits present several interesting aspects of the ambulatory payment classification (APC). For the most part, APCs follow the CPT coding rules as set forth by the AMA. However, for medical visits, hospitals have been able to develop their own criteria for assigning E/M codes that determine the level of the visit. In addition, hospitals do not follow the same guidelines as physicians (Schraffenberger and Kuehn 2011, 206).

370. **d**   In the abdomen, peritoneum, and omentum subsection, the exploratory laparotomy is a separate procedure and should not be reported when it is part of a larger procedure. The code of 49000 is often used incorrectly because laparotomy is the approach to many abdominal surgeries. The code 58720 includes bilateral and so modifier 50 is not necessary (Huey 2021, 151–152).

371. **d**   Codes for symptoms, signs, and ill-defined conditions are not to be used as the principal diagnosis when a related definitive diagnosis has been established. The flank pain would not be coded because it is a symptom of the calculus. For the ICD-10-PCS procedure code, a dilation procedure was performed using a stent inserted using ureteroscopy, so 0T788DZ is the correct code. The Section is Medical and Surgical—character 0; Body System is Urinary System—character T; Root Operation is Dilation—character 7; Body Part is Ureters, Bilateral—character 8; Approach—via Natural or Artificial Opening Endoscopic—character 8; Device—Intraluminal Device—character D; and No Qualifier—character Z (Schraffenberger and Palkie 2022, 35; Kuehn and Jorwic 2021, 109–110).

372. **c**   The National Correct Coding Initiative (NCCI or CCI) edits also apply to the APC system. The main purpose of CCI edits is to prohibit unbundling of procedures. CCI edits are updated quarterly (Casto and White 2021, 216–217).

373. **c**   Main term for diagnosis: Cystitis; subterm: chronic N30.20 is the correct code. For the ICD-10-PCS procedure code, an excision procedure was performed, so 0TBB8ZX is the correct code. The Section is Medical and Surgical—character 0; Body System is Urinary System—character T; Root Operation is Excision—character B; Body Part is Bladder—character B; Approach—via Natural or Artificial Opening Endoscopic—character 8, No Device—character Z, and the procedure was for diagnostic reasons—character X (Schraffenberger and Palkie 2022, 43–44, 469–470; Kuehn and Jorwic 2021, 72–73).

374. **b**   Code 99212 is used because the examination is medically appropriate and the medical decision-making is straightforward (Huey 2021, 338–339).

375. **b**   Main term: Hysteroscopy; lysis; adhesions. It should be noted that a surgical laparoscopy always includes a diagnostic laparoscopy (Huey 2021, 24, 174).

376. **c**   Main term for diagnosis: Incontinence, subterm: stress N39.3 is the correct code. For the ICD-10-PCS procedure code a reposition procedure was performed, 0TSD0ZZ is the correct code. The Section is Medical and Surgical—character 0; Body System is Urinary System—character T; Root Operation is Reposition—character S; Body Part is Urethra—character D; Approach—Open—character 0; No Device—character Z; and No Qualifier—character Z (Schraffenberger and Palkie 2022, 43–44; Kuehn and Jorwic 2021, 363–364).

377. a Utilization review (UR) is the process of determining whether the healthcare provided to a specific patient is necessary. Preestablished objective screening criteria are used as the basis of UR, which is performed according to time frames specified in the organization's UM plan (Miller 2020, 55).

378. c The three steps in medical necessity and utilization review are clinical review, peer review, and appeals consideration (Casto and White 2021, 29).

379. a Complications and comorbidities (CCs) and major complications and comorbidities (MCCs) also play a part in determining the Medicare severity diagnosis-related group (MS-DRG). CCs and MCCs are additional, or secondary, diagnoses that ordinarily extend the length of stay. A complication is a secondary condition that arises during hospitalization; comorbidity is one that exists at the time of admission. CCs affect many but not all MS-DRG categories. MS-DRGs are often found in sets of two or three depending on whether CCs or MCCs affect the DRG assignment. In such groupings, a case with a CC would represent a higher severity level and thus would result in a higher payment than a case without a CC. A case with an MCC would be an even higher level of severity and would pay more than a case with a CC (Gordon, M. L. 2020, 493).

380. d Medical necessity review is a cost control method to evaluate the need for and the intensity of the service prior to it being provided. Services that are cosmetic, elective, and investigational are much less likely to be considered medically necessary. Standard of care for health condition would be much more likely to be considered medically necessary (Casto and White 2021, 28–29).

381. b Discounting applies to multiple surgical procedures that have a payment status T indictor and are performed during the same operative session. For discounted procedures, the full ambulatory payment classification (APC) rate is paid for the surgical procedure with the highest rate, and other surgical procedures performed at the same time are reimbursed at 50 percent of the APC rate (Casto and White 2021, 110).

382. b An Advance Beneficiary Notice (ABN) should be provided to a patient when a service is not considered medically necessary, indicating that Medicare might not pay and that the patient may be responsible for the entire charge (Schraffenberger and Kuehn 2011, 396).

383. b Sometimes facilities adopt a bill hold policy. This policy dictates a waiting period between the patient's discharge date and claim submission (dropping the bill) (Schraffenberger and Kuehn 2011, 460).

384. a ICD-10-CM Coding Guideline I.C.15.a.4 states in the instances when a patient is admitted to a hospital for complications of pregnancy during one trimester and remains in the hospital into a subsequent trimester, the trimester character for the antepartum complication code should be assigned on the basis of the trimester the complication developed, not the trimester of the discharge (Schraffenberger and Palkie 2022, 491–492).

385. c Each diagnosis-related group (DRG) is assigned a relative weight (RW). The RW is a multiplier that determines reimbursement. For example, a DRG with a relative weight of 2.0000 would pay twice as much as a DRG with a RW of 1.0000 (Schraffenberger and Kuehn 2011, 201).

386. a Case-mix index is a weighted average of the sum of the relative weights (RWs) of all patients treated during a specified time period (Casto and White 2021, 227–228).

387. c Retrospective utilization review is conducted after the patient has been discharged. Retrospective review examines the medical necessity of the services provided to the patient while in the hospital (Gordon, M. L. 2020, 490).

388. b Coding professionals should be evaluated at least quarterly, with appropriate training needs identified, facilitated, and reassessed over time. Only through this continuous process of evaluation can data quality and integrity be accurately measured and ensured (Schraffenberger and Kuehn 2011, 353).

389. c QIOs are currently under contract with CMS to perform a Hospital Payment Monitoring Program. This program targets specific DRGs and discharges that have been identified as high risk for payment errors. The high-risk hospital specific data are identified in an electronic report called Program for Evaluating Payment Patterns Electronic Report (PEPPER) (Schraffenberger and Kuehn 2011, 32).

390. d Facilities may design the CDI program based on several different models. Improvement work can be done with retrospective record review and queries, with concurrent record review and queries, or with concurrent coding. Staffing models may include the involvement of the CDS discussed previously or could be done by enhancing the role of the utilization review staff or case managers or a combination of these models. Retrospective review of all query opportunities for the year would help to validate the effectiveness of the new program (Schraffenberger and Kuehn 2011, 363).

391. c The last component of the revenue cycle is reconciliation and collections. The healthcare facility uses the EOB, MSN, and RA to reconcile accounts. These are monitored in the claims reconciliation and collections area of the revenue cycle (Casto and White 2021, 173–174).

392. b An overpayment occurs when a facility receives higher reimbursement than the facility deserves. One example of this is when a facility submits two or more claims for the same service (Foltz and Lankisch 2020, 500).

393. d The data elements collected during the audit vary based on the audit objective. As in this example, auditing a claim for healthcare services in the emergency department could consider the following areas: procedures that are reported at the appropriate level, claims are not submitted more than once, or documentation supports services reported on the claim. Patient satisfaction with their services would not be an area of claim audit (Foltz and Lankisch 2020, 513–514).

394. b Every organization should apply the same criteria for high-quality clinical documentation to the recording of clinical documentation improvement (CDI) program activities (queries and case notes) as it does to the review of clinical documentation. Maintaining thorough query documentation is necessary for compliance purposes (Hess 2015, 241–242).

395. b Healthcare organizations should keep detailed query data. There should be documented evidence of all queries the clinical documentation improvement (CDI) specialists ask, to whom they direct queries, the clinical documentation or information supporting the query, and responses to queries. Detailed query documentation can also protect the hospital when against claims from physicians about leading queries (Hess 2015, 209).

396. a Patients should review and monitor the information found within their explanation of benefits (EOBs). Patients should not assume that their healthcare services have been accurately submitted to and paid by their insurance companies as claims submission is an error-prone process (Casto and White 2021, 172–173).

397. **b** Risk pool is a group of individual entities, such as individuals, employers, or associations, who have a similar risk of loss and whose healthcare costs are combined for evaluating financial history and estimating future costs (Casto and White 2021, 7).

398. **c** A provider may choose to accept assignment, meaning payment is based on a fee schedule, a list of services and the amount that the healthcare insurance plan will pay for healthcare claims. The provider will accept the amount paid as payment in full for the service, as opposed to balance billing where the provider charges the patient for the remainder of the costs not paid by the insurance plan (Gordon, M. L. 2020, 478).

399. **a** In case-rate methodology, the third-party payer reimburses the provider one amount for the entire visit or encounter regardless of the number of services or the length of encounter. Memorial Hospital will receive $28,500 for each admission. Case rate is a prospective reimbursement methodology. The reimbursement rate does not increase or decrease based on actual charges or actual cost of care (Casto and White 2021, 55).

400. **d** A query is appropriate to clear up ambiguous documentation, to clarify incomplete documentation and to address conflicting documentation between two providers. It is not appropriate to query a physician to question why they would document a condition (Brinda 2020, 186).

401. **a** In a global payment method the third-party payer makes a combined payment to cover the services of multiple providers, typically physicians, who are treating a single episode-of-care (Casto and White 2021, 56).

402. **d** The CC/MCC capture rate is 57.1 percent. Calculation $(15 / 70) \times 100 = 21.4\%$; $(25 / 70) \times 100 = 35.7\%$; $21.4\% + 35.7\% = 57.1\%$ (Casto and White 2021, 188–189).

403. **b** A party is an entity that receives, renders, or pays for health services. The first party is the patient or guarantor, such as the parent, responsible for the patient's health costs (Casto and White 2021, 8).

404. **c** A party is an entity that receives, renders, or pays for health services. The second party is the provider, so called because they provide healthcare. The provider may be a physician, clinic, hospital, nursing home, or other healthcare entity rendering care (Casto and White 2021, 8).

405. **a** A key performance indicator (KPI) is a quantifiable measure used to evaluate the success of an organization, employee, and the like in meeting objectives of performance. The coding manager can develop a coding dashboard to monitor and assess KPIs for their unit. The case-mix index is a KPI to measure the effectiveness of coding management (Casto and White 2021, 187).

406. **d** The CDI professional may review the record multiple times throughout the patient admission depending on the admission length of stay. When the length of stay is long enough for multiple reviews, all three of these functions are repeated multiple times: review–query–educate, repeat (Casto and White 2021, 192).

407. **c** The review rate is the total discharges available to review divided by the number of discharges to review by a CDI specialist. This is calculated as $174 / 215 \times 100 = 80.9\%$ (Casto and White 2021, 195).

408. **a** Adjudication is a back-end process of the revenue cycle. Adjudication is the determination of the reimbursement amount based on the beneficiary's insurance plan benefits (Casto and White 2021, 170–171).

409. **b**   The New Technology section contains codes for services that are new to ICD-10-PCS or that capture services not routinely captured in ICD-10-PCS that have been presented for public comment at the Coordination and Maintenance Committee Meeting. These codes may be deleted in future years, after they have served their purpose, and may or may not be recreated into the body of ICD-10-PCS at a later date (Kuehn and Jorwic 2021, 505).

410. **c**   On the CMS-1500 all procedures must be linked to one of the diagnoses listed in box 21. Linking is the assignment of diagnosis codes to individual line items (1 through 4) on a CMS-1500 claim form to cross-reference the procedure to the diagnosis code, establishing the medical necessity of the procedure (Huey 2021, 385, 512).

411. **d**   A code from category Y93, Activity code, is used to describe the activity of the patient at the time of injury or other health condition occurred. An activity code is used only once, at the initial encounter for treatment. Only one code from Y93 should be recorded on a health record (Schraffenberger and Palkie 2022, 656).

412. **d**   Electronic claims are sent electronically to the insurance payer directly or through an organization known as a clearinghouse. The electronic claims clearinghouse processes claims from multiple healthcare organizations to many insurance companies (Huey 2021, 384).

413. **c**   The physician clarification impact rate is the number of clarifications placed by a CDI intervention that had an impact on the MS-DRG assignment. This is calculated as 21 clarifications that impacted MS-DRG assignment / 35 requests sent to physicians for clarification in severity $\times$ 100 = 60% (Casto and White 2021, 195).

414. **c**   The usual and customary (U/C) fee profile concept is based on both the usual fee submitted by the provider for that code and the area customary fee for that code. Many large insurers maintain a database of the charges submitted for certain procedures by the physician over time. This database maintains the average charges that become the provider's fee profile. Math: $8.25 $\times$ 10 = $82.50; $8.75 $\times$ 20 = $175.00; $9.25 $\times$ 100 = $925.00; $82.50 + $175.00 + $925.00 = $1182.50; $1182.50 / 130 claims = $9.096 rounded to $9.10 (Huey 2021, 366–367).

415. **d**   The insurance company receives a premium in return for assuming the insureds' exposure to risk or loss (Casto and White 2021, 7).

416. **a**   Current Procedural Terminology (CPT) is a coding system used to report diagnostic and surgical services and procedures that are provided to patients. The CPT coding system is used by physicians to report services and procedures performed in the hospital inpatient and outpatient setting, and by facilities for outpatient services and procedure (Casto and White 2021, 158).

417. **d**   Healthcare fraud is the intentional deception or misrepresentation that an individual knows (or should know) to be false, or does not believe to be true, and makes, knowing the deception could result in some unauthorized benefit to himself or some other person(s). Unnecessary costs to a program, in and of itself, would not be healthcare fraud, there would need to be some intentional deception for it to be considered fraud (Foltz and Lankisch 2020, 500).

418. **b**   The U.S. Federal Sentencing Guidelines outline seven steps as the hallmark of an effective program to prevent and detect violations of law. These seven steps were the basis for the OIG's recommendations regarding the fundamental elements of an effective compliance program (Bowman 2017, 463).

419. **b**   The OIG has outlined seven elements as the minimum necessary for a comprehensive compliance program. One of the seven elements is the maintenance of a process, such as a hotline, to receive complaints and the adoption of procedures to protect the anonymity of complainants and to protect whistleblowers from retaliation (Foltz and Lankisch 2020, 504, 511).

420. **b**   Fraudulent billing practices represent a major compliance risk for healthcare organizations. High-risk billing practices include billing for noncovered services, altered claim forms, duplicate billing, misrepresentation of facts on a claim form, failing to return overpayments, unbundling, billing for medically unnecessary services, overcoding and upcoding, billing for items or services not rendered, and false cost reports (Bowman 2017, 440–441).

421. **d**   The Office of the Inspector General (OIG) continues to issue compliance program guidance for various types of healthcare organizations. The OIG website posts the documents that most healthcare organizations need to develop fraud and abuse compliance plans (Casto and White 2021, 201).

422. **d**   In conjunction with the corporate compliance officer, the health information manager should provide education and training related to the importance of complete and accurate coding, documentation, and billing on an annual basis. Technical education for all coding professionals should be provided. Documentation education is also part of compliance education. A focused effort should be made to provide documentation education to the medical staff (Schraffenberger and Kuehn 2011, 386–387).

423. **b**   The Medicare Integrity Program was established under the HIPAA legislation to battle healthcare fraud and abuse. Not only did Medicare continue to review provider claims for fraud and abuse, but the focus expanded to cost reports, payment determinations, and the need for ongoing compliance education (Casto and White 2021, 201–202).

424. **d**   Insufficient documentation in any setting can have a negative impact on compliance and reimbursement. The Comprehensive Error Rate Testing (CERT) program measures improper payments in various healthcare settings for Medicare. Assignment of improper payment categories may occur when physician offices have insufficient documentation to meet medical necessity. To determine the causes of insufficient documentation the coding supervisor should conduct a root cause analysis (Casto and White 2021, 203–204).

425. **b**   Medicare defines fraud as an intentional representation that an individual knows to be false or does not believe to be true, knowing that the representation could result in some unauthorized benefit to himself or herself or some other person. Disregard for official coding guidelines would be considered fraud (Casto and White 2021, 200).

426. **d**   In Medicare, the most common forms of fraud and abuse include billing for services not furnished; misrepresenting the diagnosis to justify payment; soliciting, offering, or receiving a kickback; unbundling; falsifying certificates of medical necessity; and billing for a service not furnished as billed, known as upcoding (Casto and White 2021, 200).

427. **d**   The policies and procedures section of a coding compliance plan should include physician query process, coding diagnosis not supported by health documentation, upcoding, correct use of encoder software, unbundling, coding health records without complete documentation, assignment of discharge destination codes, and complete process for using scrubber software. Utilization review would not be part of the policies and procedures section of a Coding Compliance Plan (Casto and White 2021, 189–190).

428. **c** The provider will be notified of RAC determination in a demand letter, which includes the providers identification, reason for the review, list of claims, reasons for any denials, and amount of the overpayment for each claim. The demand letter is the equivalent of a denial letter (Foltz and Lankisch 2020, 507–508).

429. **a** Healthcare fraud is defined as an intentional representation that an individual knows to be false or does not believe to be true, knowing that the representation could result in some unauthorized benefit to himself or herself or some other person. An example of fraud is billing for a service that was not furnished. The other three options are acceptable practices for healthcare organizations to use to effectively manage their revenue cycles (Casto and White 2021, 200).

430. **c** Risk management programs have three functions: risk identification and analysis, loss prevention and reduction, and claims management (Carter and Palmer 2020, 572).

431. **b** Most quality improvement methodologies recognize that the organization must identify and continuously monitor the important organizational and patient-focused functions that they perform. The first step in this process is to identify performance measures (Shaw and Carter 2019, 40–41).

432. **c** The formulary is composed of medications used for commonly occurring conditions or diagnoses treated in the healthcare organization. Organizations accredited by the Joint Commission are required to maintain a formulary and document that they review it at least annually for a medication's continued safety and efficacy (Shaw and Carter 2019, 221).

433. **c** Incident reports involving patient care are not created to treat the patient, but rather to provide a basis for investigating the incident. From an evidentiary standpoint, incident reports should not be placed in a patient's health record, nor should the record refer to an incident report (Klaver 2017a, 90).

434. **c** Spoliation is a legal concept applicable to both paper and electronic records. When evidence is destroyed that relates to a current or pending civil or criminal proceeding, it is reasonable to infer that the party had a consciousness of guilt or another motive to avoid the evidence (Klaver 2017a, 87).

435. **b** All individuals whose information has been breached must be notified without unreasonable delay, and not more than 60 days, by first-class mail or a faster method (such as telephone) if there is the potential for imminent misuse. If 500 or more individuals are affected, they must be individually notified immediately and media outlets must be used as a notification mechanism as well. The Secretary of HHS must specifically be notified of the breach (Rinehart-Thompson 2020b, 271).

436. **c** Each of these percentages should be tracked within the first few months of program operation. The target percentage may need adjustment over time as the CDS staff members become more familiar with their responsibilities and physician documentation improves. These percentages are record review rate, physician query rate, and query agreement rate (Hess 2015, 174–175).

437. **a** Codes are used to determine reimbursement; therefore code assignment is critical. Assigning the incorrect codes with the intent of receiving more money is fraudulent. The coding supervisor should regularly compare assigned codes to health record documentation to ensure compliance (Foltz and Lankisch 2020, 514).

438. c Productivity is defined as a unit of performance defined by management in quantitative standards. Productivity allows organizations to measure how well the organization converts input into output or labor into a product or service. 20 records per day × 5 days × 4 weeks = 400 records required to be coded. Coding professional 1 coded 400 records; coding professional 2 coded 405 records; coding professional 3 coded 345 records; coding professional 4 coded 400 records (White 2020, 156).

439. a Calling out patients' names in a physician office is an incidental disclosure because it occurs as part of office operations. It is permitted as long as the information disclosed is the minimum necessary (Rinehart-Thompson 2020b, 268).

440. c Waste is the overutilization or inappropriate utilization of services and misuse of resources, and typically is not a criminal or intentional act. Waste includes practice like over prescribing and ordering tests inappropriately (Foltz and Lankisch 2020, 501).

441. d It is imperative that all staff be trained in compliance policies, procedures, and standards of conduct as it applies to their position in the organization. This training should occur, at a minimum, in their initial orientation training and on an annual basis (Foltz and Lankisch 2020, 511).

442. a Organizations must perform internal monitoring as part of an effective compliance plan. These organizations must be diligent to ensure compliance with policies and procedures, such as through the use of audits and data analysis (Foltz and Lankisch 2020, 511).

443. c Although text messaging is often used in healthcare, it presents privacy and security risks. One best practice for text messaging in healthcare is to use encryption during transmission (Rinehart-Thompson 2018, 170).

444. c Because of compliance concerns, such as cutting and pasting documentation in the EHR, it is essential to ensure that a member of the compliance team is involved in the entire EHR implementation process, as well as the part of the process involving clinical documentation practice (Hess 2015, 269).

445. d Compliance is the process of establishing an organizational culture that promotes the prevention, detection, and resolution of instances of conduct that do not conform to federal, state, or private payer healthcare program requirements or the healthcare organization's ethical and business policies. In other words, compliance actively prevents fraud and abuse (Foltz and Lankisch 2020, 501).

446. b External audits are conducted by accreditation, insurance companies, or other organizations monitoring the healthcare provider for compliance with their standards and regulations. In this scenario, the Joint Commission is performing an external audit to determine compliance with Joint Commission standards regarding patients' rights (Foltz and Lankisch 2020, 517).

447. c Clinical documentation improvement (CDI) should be part of the organizational compliance program. The goal of a CDI compliance review is to monitor compliant query generation and physician responses (Hess 2015, 219).

448. a The Recovery Audit Contractor (RAC) program is a governmental program whose goal is to identify improper payments made on claims of healthcare services provided to Medicare beneficiaries. Improper payments may be overpayments or underpayments. Automated reviews are performed electronically rather than by humans. A software program analyzes claims data to identify improper payments (Casto and White 2021, 206).

449. **d** Health information can be threatened by humans as well as by natural and environmental factors. Threats posed by humans can be either unintentional or intentional. Threats to health information can result in compromised integrity (that is, alteration of information, either intentional or unintentional), theft (intentional by nature), loss (unintentional) or intentional misplacement, other wrongful uses or disclosures (either intentional or unintentional), and destruction (intentional or unintentional) (Rinehart-Thompson 2018, 152–153).

450. **c** One of the key components of the False Claims Act is *qui tam*. *Qui tam* is the whistleblower provisions of the False Claims Act—private persons, known as relators, may enforce the Act by filing a complaint, under seal, alleging fraud committed against the government. For example, if a coding professional is told to assign codes in violation of coding rules, then he or she can report the facility for fraud (Foltz and Lankisch 2020, 504).

451. **a** The Anti-Kickback Statute dictates that physicians cannot receive money or other benefits for referring patients to a healthcare facility. In this example, a hospital cannot give a physician $100 for every patient referred to the hospital for care (Foltz and Lankisch 2020, 504).

452. **d** Drug diversion is the removal of a medication from its usual stream of preparation, dispensing, and administration by personnel involved in those steps in order to use or sell the medication in nonhealthcare settings. An individual might take the medication for personal use, to sell on the street, to sell directly to a user as a dealer, or to sell to others who will redistribute for the diverting individual (Shaw and Carter 2019, 227–228).

453. **d** The situation presented was a near miss as it did not affect the outcome, but if the wrong drug were to have been administered before the error was caught, it had the change of being a serious adverse event. Near misses include occurrences that do not necessarily affect an outcome, but if they were to recur, they would carry significant chance of being a serious adverse event. Near misses fall under the definition of a sentinel event but are not reviewable by the Joint Commission under its current sentinel event policy. Near misses are a valuable tool for evaluation of processes and procedures, especially in high-risk or high-volume areas of facilities (Shaw and Carter 2019, 199).

454. **a** Progress, response, and changes to the patient's condition must be documented. All health records should be completely legible and accessible to patient and present diagnosis information. These are all required elements of the Medicare Conditions of Participation. Physician inclusion of vaccination records is not mandated (Hess 2015, 7).

455. **b** A cause-and-effect diagram is an investigational technique that facilitates the identification of the various factors that contribute to a problem (Carter and Palmer 2020, 565).

456. **a** The clinical documentation improvement (CDI) manager should coordinate a feedback loop with functional managers that involve reporting data from the department to CDI and then from CDI back to the department. The three areas for CDI best practices include operationalizing feedback loops with denials management, compliance, and HIM (Hess 2015, 242).

457. **d** If a patient receives a Receipt of Breach Notice from a healthcare organization it indicates that the patient's protected health information was involved in a data breach (Hamilton 2020, 667).

458. **d** A security breach of PHI has occurred in this scenario because the business office provided the patient with not only her information on the remittance advice, but also that of 10 other patients (Hamilton 2020, 669–670).

459. c   There are a number of benefits of a coding compliance plan including the retention of a high standard of coding (Foltz and Lankisch 2020, 518).

460. a   HIM professionals should be guided by the AHIMA Code of Ethics in making ethical decisions that relate to the HIM profession. In this situation, Joan and Nancy should contact AHIMA and report the abuse (Hamilton 2020, 666).

461. d   Most audits should identify some issues, either operational or compliance, in the clinical documentation improvement (CDI) process, even if they are minor issues. An organization needs to develop a corrective action plan for any identified issues (Hess 2015, 214).

462. a   A complete history and physical report represents the attending physician's assessment of the patient's current health status, and accreditation standards require it to be completed within 24 hours of admission. In this case, the HIM manager should provide the chief of surgery with information on noncompliant physicians and work together with the chief of surgery to resolve this issue (Brickner 2020a, 97).

463. b   A feedback loop between clinical documentation improvement (CDI) and health information management (HIM) should be in place as a best practice. It is necessary to ensure the CDI manager works directly with the HIM manager to obtain data about retrospective physician queries (Hess 2015, 245).

464. b   One of the information governance principles is compliance. This principle creates a process for ensuring that all the information meets requirements of appropriate laws, regulations, standards, and organizational policies (Brinda 2020, 169).

465. a   The coding compliance plan should include expectations for coding quality as one of the components of the plan (Foltz and Lankisch 2020, 518).

466. c   By reviewing all the ICD-10-CM diagnosis codes assigned to explain the reasons the services were provided (Schraffenberger and Palkie 2022, 726).

467. c   Based on the data provided in chart analysis accuracy report, only two analysts are in compliance for all four quarters of the fiscal year—John and Sue. The other analysts have one or more quarters in which they are not meeting the standard (Prater 2020, 628).

468. b   Based on the data provided in the chart analysis accuracy report, Barb has not met the compliance standard in any of the last four quarters. She also is not showing a pattern of improvement overall based on the data. Although Cathy is also not meeting the standard each quarter, she is showing improvement through the year (Prater 2020, 628).

469. a   Performance measurement compare outcomes to the established performance standards and results are typically expressed in quantifiable terms, such as rates. These are then used to determine compliance. In this instance the standard was that all patients would receive the EKG within 10 minutes of arrival. Because only 57.1% received the EKG, the facility is not in compliance with their standard (Prater 2020, 628).

470. **d** In conjunction with the corporate compliance officer, the health information manager should provide education and training related to the importance of complete and accurate coding, documentation, and billing on an annual basis. Technical education for all coding professionals should be provided. Documentation education is also part of compliance education. A focused effort should be made to provide documentation education to the medical staff. Coding is based primarily on physician documentation, so nursing staff would not be included in the education process (Foltz and Lankisch 2020, 518–519).

471. **a** Risk determination considers how likely is it that a particular threat will actually occur and, if it does occur, how great its impact or severity will be. Risk determination quantifies an organization's threats and enables it to both prioritize its risks and appropriately allocate its limited resources (namely, people, time, and money) accordingly (Rinehart-Thompson 2018, 158–159).

472. **c** The CPT code book and codes are updated annually, with additions, revisions, and deletions becoming effective on January 1st of each year. The new edition should be purchased every year to ensure accurate coding. Healthcare providers are expected to begin using the newest edition for encounters on January 1st each year. In this scenario, the department had not updated the chargemaster with the new CPT codes and were experiencing claims denials based on not monitoring these changes for accurate implementation (Smith 2021, 2)

473. **a** When writing queries, healthcare organizations must ensure they are not leading physicians to document a particular response, but rather requesting clarification or additional specifications in order to be compliant. This query is a leading query and is noncompliant (Brinda 2020, 186–187).

474. **b** The Exclusions Program is a database of individuals and healthcare organizations that are not permitted to participate in or receive payment from any federal healthcare program due to past healthcare-related crimes they committed against the federal government (Foltz and Lankisch 2020, 505).

475. **d** Compliance programs should include, when applicable, the following seven elements: policies and procedures; education and training of all employees on compliance; follow-up on all potential risk factors that may lead to an investigation; assurance that proper procedures and regulations are being followed in relation to submission of charges to health plans; principles of conduct; designation of a compliance officer or contact; and internal monitoring and auditing. Physician offices need to look at their high-risk areas such as coding, billing, documentation, and processes (workflow) (Huey 2021, 433–434).

476. **b** Authorship is the origin of recorded information that is attributed to a specific individual or entity. Electronic tools make it easier to copy and paste documentation from one record to another or to pull information forward from a previous visit, someone else's records, or other sources either intentionally or inadvertently. The ability to copy and paste entries leads to a record where a clinician may, upon signing the documentation, unwittingly swear to the accuracy and comprehensiveness of substantial amounts of duplicated, inapplicable, misleading, or erroneous information (Amatayakul 2017, 505).

477. **a** RACs conduct three types of audits: automated reviews, semi-automated reviews, and complex reviews. An automated review occurs when an RAC makes a claim determination at the system level without a human review of the health record, such as data mining. Errors found must be clearly noncovered services or incorrect applications of coding rules and must be supported by Medicare policy, approved article, or coding guidance (Foltz and Lankisch 2020, 507).

478. d   The three categories used by HHS in fighting fraud and abuse are reasonable cause, reasonable diligence, and overpayment (Foltz and Lankisch 2020, 505–506).

479. c   The data elements collected during the audit vary based on the audit objective. As in this example, auditing a claim for correct coding assignment should consider the following areas: procedures are reported at the appropriate level, claims are not submitted more than once, documentation supports services reported on the claim, and claim provides enough information for accurate code assignment. In this instance, the age is not included in the information (Foltz and Lankisch 2020, 513–514).

480. d   The focus on high dollar discharges reduced the number of accounts being released for billing and consequently the billing staff was left with limited claims to process. This disruption in the HIM workflow created a negative impact on billing that was not anticipated by the HIM director. Maintaining standards of compliance for workflow and understanding the impact on other areas of the organization must be understood (Gordon, L. L. 2020a, 536).

481. d   When writing queries, healthcare organizations must ensure they are not leading physicians to document a particular response, but rather requesting clarification or additional specifications in order to be compliant. This is an example of a compliant yes or no query resolving conflicting practitioner documentation (Brinda 2020, 186–187).

482. c   Every healthcare organization should have a written compliance plan to actively prevent fraud and abuse (Foltz and Lankisch 2020, 511).

483. d   One of the information governance principles is transparency. This stipulates that documentation related to an organization's IG initiatives be available to its workforce and other appropriate interested parties, according to the principle (Brinda 2020, 169).

484. a   Fraud is when someone intentionally executes or attempts to execute a scheme to obtain money or property of any healthcare benefit program. Abuse occurs when healthcare providers or suppliers perform actions that directly or indirectly result in unnecessary costs to any healthcare benefit program. Examples of fraud include the following: billing for services not provided to the patient; falsely documenting in medical records such as documenting a higher severity of diagnosis or completely falsifying diagnoses; directing others to falsely document or bill; or paying for referrals of federal program beneficiaries (Foltz and Lankisch 2020, 500).

485. b   A provider who intentionally fails to comply with or is acting with indifference to the HIPAA law is considered to be engaging in willful neglect (Foltz and Lankisch 2020, 506).

486. a   Upcoding is the practice of assigning diagnostic or procedural codes that results in higher payment rates than the codes that actually reflect the services provided to patients (Foltz and Lankisch 2020, 500).

487. c   The designation of POA be established for the principal and secondary diagnosis is not a factor in determining medical necessity (Schraffenberger and Palkie 2022, 726).

488. d   Staffing levels for scanning and indexing processes can be determined based on productivity standards. In this situation, each clinic visit represents a patient record that will need to be retrieved (or pulled) and stored (filed back), $8000 / 1600 = 5$; $8000 / 750 = 10.67$; $5 + 10.67 = 15.67$ hours per day rounded to 16 hours per day (White 2020, 156).

489. a   385 charts per week / 5 days / 27 standard charts per day = 2.85 (White 2020, 156).

490. **c** Coding productivity is measured by two indicators of a coding professional's skill are the types of errors he or she makes and the speed at which he or she can work (White 2020, 156–157).

491. **c** Quality coding is an important component of coding compliance. Standards for coding accuracy should be as close to 100 percent as possible (Foltz and Lankisch 2020, 518; White 2020, 156–157).

492. **c** A policy is a statement that describes general guidelines that direct behavior or direct and constrain decision-making in the organization (Gordon, L. L. 2020a, 532).

493. **c** According to the Department of Labor, the FMLA covers employees of a public agency or private firm employing 50 or more employees who work in 20 or more weeks of a calendar year; eligible employees must have worked for their employer for at least 12 months. Gender is not a consideration (Prater 2020, 614).

494. **c** In this situation, the smaller hospital should obtain a business associate agreement with the facility providing the information services (Thomason 2013, 25).

495. **c** The HIPAA Privacy Rule intent is to allow an individual to obtain copies of records for a fee that is reasonable enough that an individual could pay for it. The Privacy Rule requires that the copy fee for the individual be reasonable and cost based. It can only include the costs of labor for copying and postage, when mailed. The commentary to the Privacy Rule expands upon this standard. If paper copies are made, the fee can include the cost of the paper. If electronic copies are made, the fee can include copies of the media used (Thomason 2013, 96).

496. **a** One of the ways to speed data entry is through the copy and paste functions. Data from one patient's health record can be copied and pasted into another patient's health record or data from the same patient's previous hospitalization may be moved to their current hospitalization. Although this function speeds data entry, there is a data quality risk if the information copied may not completely apply to the patient's care. When this happens, the patient's health record contains erroneous information that can impact the quality of care (Sayles and Kavanaugh-Burke 2021, 29).

497. **b** Change management is the formal process of introducing change, getting it adopted, and diffusing it throughout the organization (Gordon, L. L. 2020b, 590).

498. **a** Flowcharts help all the team members understand the process in the same way. The work involved in developing the flowchart allows the team to thoroughly understand every step in the process as well as the sequence of steps. The flowchart provides a visual picture of each decision point and each event that must be completed. It readily points out places where there are redundancy and complex and problematic areas (Carter and Palmer 2020, 563).

499. **a** The first step in benchmarking is to determine the performance measure to be studied and what is to be accomplished. Once a benchmark for a performance measure is determined, analyzing data collection results becomes more meaningful (Shaw and Carter 2019, 42).

500. **a** Individual audit results by the coding professional may identify that certain coding professionals are ready to be cross-trained in another category of coding. Regardless of the corrective actions taken, the results should become part of each employee's performance evaluation (Schraffenberger and Kuehn 2011, 324).

501. **b** Comparing an organization's performance to the performance of other organizations that provide the same types of service is known as benchmarking. Internal benchmarking is also important to establish a baseline for the organization to find ways to improve effectiveness. Benchmark averages can be helpful in setting productivity standards, but do not necessarily reflect variations in procedures from organization to organization. Investigating what factors may be contributing to the low productivity for this organization will give a better understanding of the variation (Shaw and Carter 2019, 42).

502. **c** The four criteria describing the basics of best practice in CDI programs are: remain constant over time; be supported by research or actual application by more than one healthcare system; affect at least two out of three management areas; and provide some measurable value to the organization (Hess 2015, 239).

503. **a** Managers must be able to report on the amount, efficiency, and quality of work being done in a unit. Employees need to know what is expected of them, and how they are doing relative to expectations. Setting performance standards and measuring performance can address the needs of both (Prater 2020, 628).

504. **c** A standard should be set that all query opportunities within a CDI program should undergo comprehensive review retrospectively at least once a year (Hess 2015, 211).

505. **b** Operational planning is the specific day-to-day tasks required in operating a healthcare organization or an HIM department. Making up the weekly work schedule would be part of operational planning (Gordon, L. L. 2020a, 534–535).

506. **a** Because the financial impact of a clinical documentation improvement (CDI) program is important and because many programs may lose their continued funding without the ability to demonstrate economic value, every organization should have a best practices approach to managing the financial measurement of its CDI program. One of these best practices is to track and report on MCC and CC capture rates across the organization and by service (Hess 2015, 251).

507. **a** Planning is the examination of the future and preparation of action strategies to attain goals of the department or healthcare facility; for example, a director in the HIM department may use the planning function to prepare for the future state of the department after the implementation of a new release of information software system installation (Gordon, L. L. 2020a, 528).

508. **c** Planned change is a formal process that is introduced methodically and is actively influenced by a manager or change agents (Kelly and Greenstone 2020, 87)

509. **d** In order to be both effective and efficient, each organization must be guided by policies and procedures that are created and specific to the organization. This includes policies and procedures regarding clinical documentation (Hess 2015, 172).

510. **a** Early adopters are a little more cautious than the innovators but these individuals are the change leaders within the organization. These individuals do not require information to change but they like to have how-to manuals and information sheets on how to participate within the change, which can be provided by the change agents. In this situation, Dr. Jones is an early adopter of the e-prescribing application (Kelly and Greenstone 2020, 84).

511. **d** HIPAA provides standards regarding administrative requirements that are important to the health information professional, including requirements for privacy training. Every member of the covered entity's workforce must be trained in PHI policies and procedures to include maintaining the privacy of patient information, upholding individual rights guaranteed by the Privacy Rule, and reporting alleged breaches and other Privacy Rule violations (Rinehart-Thompson 2020b, 273).

512. **c** A needs assessment is a procedure performed by collecting and analyzing data to determine what is required, lacking, or desired by an employee, group, or organization. A needs assessment is a process for determining how to close a learning or performance gap as it relates to jobs performed in a particular department (Kelly and Greenstone 2020, 129–130).

513. **b** When an organization compares its current performance to its own internal historical data, or uses data from similar external organizations across the country, it helps establish a benchmark, also known as a standard of performance or best practice, for a particular process or outcome (Shaw and Carter 2019, 42).

514. **d** Controlling is the function in which performance is monitored according to policies and procedures. In HIM, controlling includes monitoring the performance of employees for quality, accuracy, and timeliness of completion of duties (Gordon, L. L. 2020a, 528).

515. **b** Secondary data sources for job analysis are information obtained from subject matter experts, human resource consultants, job data banks, or competency models. The AHIMA Body of Knowledge would be considered data from subject matter experts (Kelly and Greenstone 2020, 131).

516. **d** While managing conflict, there are times when difficult or critical conversations need to take place in order for resolution to occur to move change to the next level. Poor communication creates obstacles for managing critical conversations in conflict situations. Critical or crucial conversations are about challenging issues where emotions are involved and the outcomes of the conversation have a large impact on relationships or workplace dynamics (Kelly and Greenstone 2020, 99–100).

517. **a** Managers can collect information about a job from a variety of sources. One of these is to use external sources' data for job analysis. In this scenario, Jane contacts other external sources at other facilities in order to use their information to create the scanning function requirements (Prater 2020, 617–618).

518. **b** The underlying tenet is all human beings prefer doing things that have the most meaning for themselves. When people believe change is going to be harmful to themselves or their career they are resistant to change. To overcome this resistance, leaders need to patiently sell the idea of change by educating their team and carefully disseminating information. Missing planning meetings would be perceived as being resistant to the change (Gordon, L. L. 2020b, 590).

519. **c** Work imaging occurs when the supervisor gets a snapshot of the current process and then use that data, along with benchmarking data, to establish standards for a position within their department (Schraffenberger and Kuehn 2011, 276–279).

520. **c** Managers must be able to report on the amount, efficiency, and quality of work being done in a unit. Employees need to know what is expected of them, and how they are doing relative to expectations. Setting performance standards and measuring performance can address the needs of both (Prater 2020, 628).

521. **a** Comparing an organization's performance to the performance of other organizations that provide the same types of service is known as benchmarking. Internal benchmarking is also important to establish a baseline for the organization to find ways to improve effectiveness (Shaw and Carter 2019, 42).

522. **b** Organization is coordinating all of the tasks and responsibilities of a department to guarantee the work to be accomplished is completed correctly. A director or supervisor is responsible for the decisions concerning the division of labor for the HIM department (Gordon, L. L. 2020a, 529).

523. **d** A job description, sometimes called a position description, is a written explanation of a job and the duties it entails based on information provided by the job analysis. A job description helps the human resources department, hiring manager, the employee's direct supervisor, and the employee understand the job duties and expectations (Prater 2020, 618–619).

524. **c** Classroom-based learning refers to instructor-led, face-to-face training such as traditional lectures, workshops, and seminars. This method is commonly used by managers because it is familiar and content is relatively quick, easy, and inexpensive to develop (Prater 2020, 645).

525. **d** Telecommuting, also called remote or virtual work, allows employees to use technology to perform work and link with the organization from home or another out-of-office location. The organization usually provides a computer and the required software (Prater 2020, 627).

526. **a** Performance appraisal refers to the formal system of review and evaluation methods used to assess employee and team performance. The 360 performance appraisal method utilizes team members as part of the appraisal process. Some of the pros of this method are that bias is reduced by including multiple perspectives from inside and outside the organization (that is, managers, subordinates, peers, customers; may also include self-appraisal); it is development-focused; less useful for promotion, compensation; and it emphasizes team and customer relationships (Prater 2020, 631–632).

527. **d** Performance measurement compares work outcomes to the established performance standards and results are typically expressed in quantifiable terms, such as rates. An 18% error rate on abstracting data would be indicative of a process problem in the HIM department. The other three options are process problems for other areas of the hospital (Prater 2020, 628).

528. **c** Leading is the function in which people are directed and motivated to achieve the goals of the healthcare organization. In this scenario, the HIM director is performing the leading function of management (Gordon, L. L. 2020a, 528).

529. **b** A policy is a governing principle that describe how a department or an organization is supposed to handle a specific situation or execute a specific process (Gordon, L. L. 2020a, 532).

530. **d** Turnaround time is the time between receipt of the release of information (ROI) request and when the request is sent to the requestor. The supervisor is responsible for insuring that release of information ROI turnaround times are met (Sayles 2020b, 70).

531. **a** Productivity is defined as a unit of performance defined by management in quantitative standards. Productivity allows organization to measure how well the organization converts input into output, or labor into a product or service. Most HIM departments have productivity standards in the department, such as coding, analysis, and release of information (White 2020, 156–157).

532. **c** An effective tool for planning and tracking the implementation of a project is the Gantt chart. A Gantt chart is a graphic tool used to plot tasks in project management that shows the duration of project tasks and overlapping tasks. This project management methodology is used for planning and tracking patient care processes (Shaw and Carter 2019, 369).

533. **a** Patient education and engagement, including educating patients about their consent options in health information exchange, who may release their information and how, and the significance of the consent choice, is a key component of a meaningful consent program (Sayles and Kavanaugh-Burke 2021, 269–270).

534. **c** A procedure is a document that describes the steps involved in performing a specific function that define the processes by which the policies are put into action (Gordon, L. L. 2020a, 532).

535. **d** The process to develop a strategic and operational plan begins with a SWOT (acronym for strengths, weaknesses, opportunities, and threats) analysis. In a SWOT analysis, key leadership personnel determine the strengths of the organization (what the company does well), the weaknesses (needs for improvement), and establishes future opportunities (and evaluates threats to those opportunities). This scenario is an example of threat in the SWOT analysis (Gordon, L. L. 2020a, 535).

536. **a** Policies are the principles describing how a department or an organization will handle a specific situation or execute a specific process. They are clear, simple statements of how an HIM department will conduct its services, actions, or business; and a set of guidelines and steps to help with decision-making (Gordon, L. L. 2020a, 532).

537. **d** Competencies are "do" statements identifying measurable skills, abilities, behaviors, or other characteristics required of an individual in order to complete the work required in a successful manner. This example provides competencies for a release of information specialist (Prater 2020, 618).

538. **a** A dashboard is a management report of process measures. Dashboards can assist in measuring whether or not the program is successful. A monthly dashboard might show the number of clarifications requested by a CDI specialist that impacted a diagnosis-related group based on a benchmark (Bowe and Williamson, 2020, 367).

539. **c** Reasonable accommodations are actions taken by an employer to allow a disabled applicant or employee access to a work opportunity. The disabled person is typically expected to request the accommodation. Examples of accommodations might include altering their work schedule, or modifying office equipment or software (Prater 2020, 613).

540. **b** New employee orientation includes a group of activities to help the employee feel knowledgeable and competent. Educational programs required for employees organization-wide (such as HIPAA, privacy, and such) are part of training initiated with new employee orientation (Prater 2020, 643).

541. **b** The critical incident method is a method of performance appraisal that includes an ongoing written log of examples of an employee's job-related behavior during the appraisal period is used. It offers specific examples for development and is important that a manager documents both positive actions and negative incidents. This method can be used to supplement rating methods (Prater 2020, 632).

542. c   Performance monitoring is data driven. The organization's leadership uses the information displayed on the dashboard to guide operations and determine improvement projects. Having real-time data in an easily assessable format like a dashboard allows leaders to keep track of high-impact, high-risk, or high-value processes and make adjustments on a daily basis if needed (Carter and Palmer 2020, 552).

543. c   A procedure is a document that describes the steps involved in performing a specific function (Gordon, L. L. 2020a, 532).

544. b   An internal analysis involves reviewing the inner working of the healthcare organization to determine strengths and weaknesses of the business practice and process. The scenario is an example of internal analysis (Gordon, L. L. 2020a, 535).

545. b   A policy is a clearly stated and comprehensive statement that establishes the parameters for decision-making and action and is the written description of the organization's formal position. Policies are developed at both the institutional and departmental levels. In both cases, policies should be consistent within the organization. They must be developed in accordance with applicable laws and reflect actual practice (Gordon, L. L. 2020a, 532).

546. d   The program evaluation and review technique (PERT) provides a structure that requires the project team to identify the order and projected duration of activities needed to complete a project. The path with the greatest total duration time is called the critical path and represents the longest amount of time required to complete the total project (Shaw and Carter 2019, 370).

547. d   Work sampling is a statistical method that reviews a select portion of tasks performed and provides baseline data for further job performance assessment. Work sampling takes into account the quantity of activities that can be completed within a certain timeframe (Kelly and Greenstone 2020, 183).

548. a   Source systems include the electronic medication administration record (EMAR), laboratory information system, radiology information system, hospital information system, nursing information systems, and more (Sayles and Kavanaugh-Burke 2021, 170).

549. d   Interoperability is the ability of different information technology systems and software applications to communicate; to exchange data accurately, effectively, and consistently; and to use the information that has been exchanged (Sayles and Kavanaugh-Burke 2021, 252).

550. c   One or more individuals in an organization normally sponsor a project. The personal commitment a sponsor brings to a project coincides with the degree of empowerment a project manager will have. Sponsorship by top leadership, therefore, must be characterized by commitment and clear articulation of expectations (Shaw and Carter 2019, 366).

RESOURCES

References

45 CFR 160.103: General Administrative Requirements: General Provisions: Definitions. 2006.

Amatayakul, M. K. 2020. Health Information Technologies. Chapter 11 in *Health Information Management Technology: An Applied Approach*, 6th ed. Edited by N. B. Sayles and L. L. Gordon. Chicago: AHIMA.

Amatayakul, M. K. 2017. *Health IT and EHRs: Principles and Practice*, 6th ed. Chicago: American Health Information Management Association.

American Health Information Management Association. 2017. *Pocket Glossary of Health Information Management and Technology*, 5th ed. Chicago: AHIMA.

Bowe, H. and L. M. Williamson. 2020. Healthcare Information. Chapter 12 in *Health Information Management Technology: An Applied Approach*, 6th ed. Edited by N. B. Sayles and L. L. Gordon. Chicago: AHIMA.

Bowman, S. 2017. Corporate Compliance. Chapter 18 in *Fundamentals of Law for Health Informatics and Information Management*, 3rd ed. Edited by M. S. Brodnik, L. A. Rinehart-Thompson, and R. B. Reynolds. Chicago: AHIMA.

Brickner, M. R. 2020a. Health Record Content and Documentation. Chapter 4 in *Health Information Management Technology: An Applied Approach*, 6th ed. Edited by N. B. Sayles and L. L. Gordon. Chicago: AHIMA.

Brickner, M. R. 2020b. Data Security. Chapter 10 in *Health Information Management Technology: An Applied Approach*, 6th ed. Edited by N. B. Sayles and L. L. Gordon. Chicago: AHIMA.

Brinda, D. 2020. Data Management. Chapter 6 in *Health Information Management Technology: An Applied Approach*, 6th ed. Edited by N. B. Sayles and L. L. Gordon. Chicago: AHIMA.

Brodnik, M. S. 2017a. Introduction to the Fundamentals of Law for Health Informatics and Information Management. Chapter 1 in *Fundamentals of Law for Health Informatics and Information Management*, 3rd ed. Edited by M. S. Brodnik, L. A. Rinehart-Thompson, and R. B. Reynolds. Chicago: AHIMA.

Brodnik, M. S. 2017b. Access, Use, and Disclosure and Release of Health Information. Chapter 15 in *Fundamentals of Law for Health Informatics and Information Management*, 3rd ed. Edited by M. S. Brodnik, L. A. Rinehart-Thompson, and R. B. Reynolds. Chicago: AHIMA.

Brodnik, M. S. 2017c. Required Reporting and Mandatory Disclosure Laws. Chapter 16 in *Fundamentals of Law for Health Informatics and Information Management*, 3rd ed. Edited by M. S. Brodnik, L. A. Rinehart-Thompson, and R. B. Reynolds. Chicago: AHIMA.

Brodnik, M. S., L. A. Rinehart-Thompson, and R. B. Reynolds. 2017. *Fundamentals of Law for Health Informatics and Information Management*, 3rd ed. Chicago: AHIMA.

Carter, D. and M. N. Palmer. 2020. Performance Improvement. Chapter 18 in *Health Information Management Technology: An Applied Approach*, 6th ed. Edited by N. B. Sayles and L. L. Gordon. Chicago: AHIMA.

Casto, A. B. and S. White. 2021. *Principles of Healthcare Reimbursement*, 7th ed. Chicago: AHIMA.

Fahrenholz, C. G. 2017. *Documentation for Health Records,* 2nd ed. Chicago: AHIMA.

Fahrenholz, C. G. 2017a. Principal and Ancillary Functions of the Healthcare Record. Chapter 3 in *Documentation for Health Records,* 2nd ed. Chicago: AHIMA.

Fahrenholz, C. G. 2017b. Documentation for Statistical Reporting and Public Health. Chapter 4 in *Documentation for Health Records,* 2nd ed. Chicago: AHIMA.

Fahrenholz, C. G. 2017c. Clinical Documentation and the Health Record. Chapter 2 in *Documentation for Health Records,* 2nd ed. Chicago: AHIMA.

Foltz, D. A. and K. M. Lankisch. 2020. Fraud and Abuse Compliance. Chapter 16 in *Health Information Management Technology: An Applied Approach*, 6th ed. Edited by N. B. Sayles and L. L. Gordon. Chicago: AHIMA.

Gordon, L. L. 2020a. Management. Chapter 17 in *Health Information Management Technology: An Applied Approach*, 6th ed. Edited by N. B. Sayles and L. L. Gordon. Chicago: AHIMA.

Gordon, L. L. 2020b. Leadership. Chapter 19 in *Health Information Management Technology: An Applied Approach*, 6th ed. Edited by N. B. Sayles and L. L. Gordon. Chicago: AHIMA.

Gordon, M. L. 2020. Revenue Management and Reimbursement. Chapter 15 in *Health Information Management Technology: An Applied Approach*, 6th ed. Edited by N. B. Sayles and L. L. Gordon. Chicago: AHIMA.

Hamilton, M. 2020. Ethical Issues in Health Information Management. Chapter 21 in *Health Information Management Technology: An Applied Approach*, 6th ed. Edited by N. B. Sayles and L. L. Gordon. Chicago: AHIMA.

Hess, P. 2015. *Clinical Documentation Improvement: Principles and Practice*. Chicago: AHIMA.

Huey, K. 2021. *Procedural Coding and Reimbursement for Physician Services: Applying Current Procedural Terminology and HCPCS, 2021*. Chicago: AHIMA.

Hunt, T. J. 2017. Clinical Documentation Improvement. Chapter 6 in *Documentation for Health Records*, 2nd ed. Chicago: AHIMA.

James, E. L. 2017. Facility-Based Long-Term Care. Chapter 12 in *Documentation for Health Records,* 2nd ed. Chicago: AHIMA.

Johns, M. 2015. *Enterprise Health Information Management and Data Governance*. Chicago: AHIMA.

Kelly, J. and P. Greenstone. 2020. *Management for the Health Information Professional*, 2nd ed. Chicago: AHIMA.

Klaver, J. C. 2017a. Evidence. Chapter 5 in *Fundamentals of Law for Health Informatics and Information Management*, 3rd ed. Edited by M. S. Brodnik, L. A. Rinehart-Thompson, and R. B. Reynolds. Chicago: AHIMA.

Klaver, J. C. 2017b. Consent to Treatment. Chapter 8 in *Fundamentals of Law for Health Informatics and Information Management*, 3rd ed. Edited by M. S. Brodnik, L. A. Rinehart-Thompson, and R. B. Reynolds. Chicago: AHIMA.

Kuehn, L. and T. M. Jorwic. 2021. *ICD-10-PCS: An Applied Approach,* 2021. Chicago: AHIMA.

Marc, D. and R. Sandefer. 2016. *Data Analytics in Healthcare Research: Tools and Strategies*. Chicago: AHIMA.

McNeill, M. H. 2020. Healthcare Statistics. Chapter 14 in *Health Information Management Technology: An Applied Approach*, 6th ed. Edited by N. B. Sayles and L. L. Gordon. Chicago: AHIMA.

Miller, K. 2020. Healthcare Delivery Systems. Chapter 2 in *Health Information Management Technology: An Applied Approach*, 6th ed. Edited by N. B. Sayles and L. L. Gordon. Chicago: AHIMA.

Prater, V. S. 2020. Human Resources Management and Professional Development. Chapter 20 in *Health Information Management Technology: An Applied Approach*, 6th ed. Edited by N. B. Sayles and L. L. Gordon. Chicago: AHIMA.

Reynolds, R. B. and M. S. Brodnik. 2017. The HIPAA Security Rule. Chapter 12 in *Fundamentals of Law for Health Informatics and Information Management*, 3rd ed. Edited by M. S. Brodnik, L. A. Rinehart-Thompson, and R. B. Reynolds. Chicago: AHIMA.

Rinehart-Thompson, L. A. 2020a. Health Law. Chapter 8 in *Health Information Management Technology: An Applied Approach*, 6th ed. Edited by N. B. Sayles and L. L. Gordon. Chicago: AHIMA.

Rinehart-Thompson, L. A. 2020b. Data Privacy and Confidentiality. Chapter 9 in *Health Information Management Technology: An Applied Approach*, 6th ed. Edited by N. B. Sayles and L. L. Gordon. Chicago: AHIMA.

Rinehart-Thompson, L. A. 2018. *Introduction to Health Information Privacy and Security,* 2nd ed. Chicago: AHIMA.

Rinehart-Thompson, L. A. 2017a. Legal Proceedings. Chapter 4 in *Fundamentals of Law for Health Informatics and Information Management*, 3rd ed. Edited by M. S. Brodnik, L. A. Rinehart-Thompson, and R. B. Reynolds. Chicago: AHIMA.

Rinehart-Thompson, L. A. 2017b. Legal Health Record: Maintenance, Content, Documentation, and Disposition. Chapter 9 in *Fundamentals of Law for Health Informatics and Information Management*, 3rd ed. Edited by M. S. Brodnik, L. A. Rinehart-Thompson, and R. B. Reynolds. Chicago: AHIMA.

Rinehart-Thompson, L. A. 2017c. HIPAA Privacy Rule: Part I. Chapter 10 in *Fundamentals of Law for Health Informatics and Information Management*, 3rd ed. Edited by M. S. Brodnik, L. A. Rinehart-Thompson, and R. B. Reynolds. Chicago: AHIMA.

Rinehart-Thompson, L. A. 2017d. HIPAA Privacy Rule: Part II. Chapter 11 in *Fundamentals of Law for Health Informatics and Information Management*, 3rd ed. Edited by M. S. Brodnik, L. A. Rinehart-Thompson, and R. B. Reynolds. Chicago: AHIMA.

Rinehart-Thompson, L. A. 2017e. Federal and State Requirements and Accreditation Guidelines. Chapter 9 in *Documentation for Health Records,* 2nd ed. Chicago: AHIMA.

Rinehart-Thompson, L. A. 2017f. Tort Law. Chapter 4 in *Fundamentals of Law for Health Informatics and Information Management*, 3rd ed. Edited by M. S. Brodnik, L. A. Rinehart-Thompson, and R. B. Reynolds. Chicago: AHIMA.

Rossiter, S. 2017. Ambulatory Care Documentation, Accreditation, Liability, and Standards. Chapter 10 in *Documentation for Health Records,* 2nd ed. Chicago: AHIMA.

Sayles, N. B. 2020a. Health Information Management Profession. Chapter 1 in *Health Information Management Technology: An Applied Approach*, 6th ed. Edited by N. B. Sayles and L. L. Gordon. Chicago: AHIMA.

Sayles, N. B. 2020b. Health Information Functions, Purpose, and Users. Chapter 3 in *Health Information Management Technology: An Applied Approach*, 6th ed. Edited by N. B. Sayles and L. L. Gordon. Chicago: AHIMA.

Sayles, N. B. and L. Gordon. 2020. *Health Information Management Technology: An Applied Approach*, 6th ed. Chicago: AHIMA.

Sayles, N. B. and L. Kavanaugh-Burke. 2021. *Introduction to Information Systems for Health Information Technology*, 4th ed. Chicago: AHIMA.

Schraffenberger, L. A. and L. Kuehn. 2011. *Effective Management of Coding Services*, 3rd ed. Chicago: AHIMA.

Schraffenberger, L. A. and B. Palkie. 2022. *Basic ICD-10-CM and ICD-10-PCS Coding, 2022*. Chicago: AHIMA.

Selman-Holman, L. 2017. Home Care and Hospice Documentation, Liability, and Standards. Chapter 13 in *Documentation for Health Records,* 2nd ed. Chicago: AHIMA.

Sharp, M. 2020. Secondary Data Sources. Chapter 7 in *Health Information Management Technology: An Applied Approach*, 6th ed. Edited by N. B. Sayles and L. L. Gordon. Chicago: AHIMA.

Shaw, P. L. and D. Carter. 2019. *Quality and Performance Improvement in Healthcare: Theory, Practice, and Management*, 7th ed. Chicago: AHIMA.

Smith, G. I. 2021. *Basic Current Procedural Terminology and HCPCS Coding, 2021*. Chicago: AHIMA.

Thomason, M. C. 2013. *HIPAA by Example: Application of Privacy Laws*, 2nd ed. Chicago: AHIMA.

White, S. 2021. *A Practical Approach to Analyzing Healthcare Data*, 4th ed. Chicago: AHIMA.

White, S. 2020. *Calculating and Reporting Healthcare Statistics*, 6th ed. Chicago: AHIMA.

Williamson, L. M. 2020. Research and Data Analysis. Chapter 13 in *Health Information Management Technology: An Applied Approach*, 6th ed. Edited by N. B. Sayles and L. L. Gordon. Chicago: AHIMA.

Formulas

Hospital Statistical Formulas Used for the RHIT Exam

Average Daily Census

$$\frac{\text{Total inpatient service for the unit for the period}}{\text{Total number of days in the period}}$$

Average Length of Stay

$$\frac{\text{Total length of stay for a given period}}{\text{Total discharges (includes deaths)}}$$

Percentage of Occupancy

$$\frac{\text{Total inpatient service days for a period}}{\text{Total inpatient bed count days in the period}} \times 100$$

Hospital Death Rate (Gross)

$$\frac{\text{Number of deaths of inpatients in period}}{\text{Number of discharges (including deaths)}} \times 100$$

Gross Autopsy Rate

$$\frac{\text{Total inpatient autopsies for a given period}}{\text{Total inpatient deaths for the period}} \times 100$$

Net Autopsy Rate

$$\frac{\text{Total inpatient autopsies for a given period}}{\text{Total inpatient deaths} - \text{unautopsied coroner's or medical examiners' cases for the same period}} \times 100$$

Hospital Autopsy Rate

$$\frac{\text{Total hospital autopsies for a given period}}{\text{Number of deaths of hospital patients whose bodies are available for hospital autopsy for the same period}} \times 100$$

Fetal Death Rate

$$\frac{\text{Total number of intermediate and/or late fetal deaths for a period}}{\text{Total number of live births} + \text{intermediate and late fetal deaths for the period}} \times 100$$

Neonatal Mortality Rate (Death Rate)

$$\frac{\text{Total number of deaths of infants from birth up to, but not including, 28 days of age for a period}}{\text{Total number of live births for the period}} \times 100$$

Maternal Mortality Rate (Death Rate)

$$\frac{\text{Total number of direct maternal deaths for a period}}{\text{Total number of maternal obstetrical discharges (including deaths) for the period}} \times 100$$

Caesarean-Section Rate

$$\frac{\text{Total number of Caesarean sections performed in a period}}{\text{Total number of deliveries in the period (including Caesarean sections)}} \times 100$$